Victorious Steps

Triumph over Diabetes through Faith and Fitness

By: Brighton Mumvuri

1

Dedication

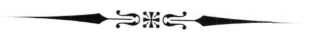

In recognition of your unwavering strength, resilience, and enduring spirit in the face of diabetes, I dedicate this book, "Victorious Steps: Triumph over Diabetes through Faith and Fitness," to each of you.

I extend my deepest gratitude to my beloved wife and family for their unwavering love, patience, and support throughout my own diabetes complications. Your strength and understanding have been my refuge in the face of adversity.

To my beloved Mother, whose enduring grace and determination have been a guiding light throughout my life, and whose own journey with diabetes has shown me the true meaning of courage.

To my brother Kudzai, a source of inspiration and strength, whose tenacity in living with diabetes serves as a powerful reminder that we can conquer any challenge life presents.

To Israel and Washington my brothers, Rosa, and Martha, my cherished sisters, who have faced the complexities of diabetes with grace and unity, demonstrating the strength of our family bond.

In loving memory of our relatives, some of whom we have lost to the relentless grip of diabetes. Your memory lives on as a reminder of the importance of our collective commitment to fighting this condition.

To all those living with diabetes, this book is a tribute to your enduring spirit and your shared journey. May it serve as a source of inspiration and guidance as we walk this path together.

To my remarkable medical team, who have stood by my side since 2007, offering expert care, guidance, and unwavering support, I am profoundly thankful for your dedication to my well-being.

My heartfelt appreciation also goes out to the National Health Service (NHS) for its commitment to providing high-quality healthcare and support to individuals living with diabetes.

With gratitude and the shared determination to overcome, I present this book as a testament to the power of unity and hope in our fight against diabetes.

Sincerely,

Brighton Mumvuri

Endorsements

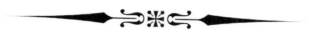

I am delighted to offer my wholehearted endorsement for "Victorious Steps" by Brighton Mumvuri. This book is a remarkable and inspirational journey that underscores the profound impact of faith, fitness, and resilience in the battle against diabetes.

Through personal experience and profound insights, Brighton Mumvuri shares a compelling narrative that not only resonates with those affected by diabetes but also provides invaluable guidance for managing this complex condition. The candid account of his own struggles and triumphs serves as a beacon of hope for anyone grappling with diabetes.

"Victorious Steps" offers practical strategies and advice to empower readers to take control of their diabetes management. The emphasis on faith and the transformative power of fitness is both refreshing and motivating. It's a testament to the resilience of the human spirit and the capacity to overcome adversity.

As a healthcare professional, I appreciate the book's emphasis on the importance of a holistic approach to diabetes management, one that encompasses physical, emotional, and spiritual well-being. It's a message that resonates deeply with the comprehensive care we aim to provide to our patients.

I wholeheartedly recommend "Victorious Steps" to anyone touched by diabetes—patients, caregivers, and healthcare providers alike. It's a powerful testament to the potential for triumph in the face of adversity, and I believe it will inspire and guide many on their journey to better health and a more fulfilling life.

Dr A Smith (London)

I am deeply privileged to provide my endorsement for "Victorious Steps" by Brighton, a book that has profoundly influenced my own path with diabetes. As both a diabetic patient and Brighton's sibling, I can unequivocally affirm the authenticity and significance of this compelling narrative.

"Victorious Steps" is not just a book; it's a lifeline for anyone facing the daily challenges of diabetes. Brighton's personal story of resilience, faith, and the transformative power of fitness resonates deeply with my own experience. His journey from struggle to triumph serves as an enduring source of inspiration for me.

What sets this book apart is its practicality. Brighton provides actionable advice, tips, and strategies for managing diabetes that have genuinely transformed my approach to this condition. From embracing a healthier lifestyle to strengthening my faith, I've found solace and hope within these pages.

As someone living with diabetes, I wholeheartedly recommend "Victorious Steps" to my fellow patients. It offers not just guidance but a sense of camaraderie—a reminder that we are not alone in this journey. Brighton's unwavering spirit and commitment to helping others shine through in every chapter.

This book is a testament to the fact that we can overcome the challenges of diabetes and live a fulfilling life. It has been an incredible source of support and motivation for me, and I believe it will be the same for many others.

Israel Mumvuri

Table of Contents

Preface

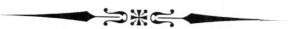

Welcome to the pages of **"Victorious Steps: Triumph over Diabetes through Faith and Fitness."** As I stand at the threshold of sharing this journey with you, I'm filled with a deep sense of purpose and gratitude. This book is a testament to the incredible power we possess within us to conquer the challenges that life presents, particularly the formidable foe of diabetes.

You might wonder what inspired me to pen this book. It's my story, a deeply personal journey through the complexities of diabetes. My narrative is not just a tale of personal triumph; it's a beacon of hope, illuminating the path to victory through my unwavering faith and the embrace of a healthier, more active lifestyle.

"Victorious Steps" isn't just about conquering diabetes; it's about embracing life with a newfound sense of purpose and empowerment. It underscores the profound connection between our physical well-being and the strength of our faith—a connection that has the potential to reshape our lives.

Throughout the pages that follow, you'll encounter my real-life story of courage, expert insights, and practical strategies that will empower you to navigate the challenges of diabetes with resilience and determination. This book is more than just information; it's a roadmap to a life where medical help, faith, fitness, and victory converge.

With each chapter, we'll take steps together, each one bringing us closer to a life of triumph. Whether you are someone living with diabetes, a caregiver, or a curious soul seeking to understand this condition better, I invite you to embark on this journey with me. Let us walk hand in hand, knowing that each page turned is a step toward a healthier, more fulfilling life.

May the stories within these pages inspire you, the knowledge empower you, and the faith strengthen you. Remember, we are not alone on this journey. "Victorious Steps" is here to guide you, support you, and remind you that, indeed, triumph over diabetes is possible.

With unwavering faith and a heart full of hope,

Brighton Mumvuri

Introduction:

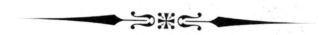

Victorious Steps: Triumph over Diabetes " - an empowering and uplifting journey of one individual's battle with diabetes and their incredible triumph through the unwavering power of faith and a dedicated fitness regime.

In this inspiring book, Brighton, a determined fighter against diabetes, bares his soul and shares his remarkable story. From a life that was sedentary and not active when he was diagnosed to the moment of diagnosis that shook his world, Brighton takes us on a deeply personal journey through the highs and lows of his fight with this relentless condition. He opens his heart, recounting the emotional struggles, the physical challenges of managing blood sugar levels, and the inspiring moments that propelled him forward. From the support of his loved ones to the camaraderie found in diabetes support groups, Brighton offers a roadmap to finding strength in community.

With unwavering faith in God as his anchor, Brighton embarks on a remarkable transformation. Through the pages of this book, he unveils the powerful role that faith and fitness played in fuelling his determination to overcome diabetes. In the face of adversity, he draws strength from his spiritual connection, finding solace and resilience in the power of prayer.

But faith and medicine alone were not the sole tools in Brighton's arsenal. Recognizing the importance of a comprehensive approach, he turned to fitness to take control of his health. Starting with a simple decision to embrace exercise on that defining moment on 27th July 2011, Brighton's journey evolved from jogging to running marathons, shedding excess weight, and reclaiming his vitality.

This book transcends being merely a personal testimony; it stands as a beacon of hope for all those wrestling with diabetes. Drawing from his own experiences, Brighton imparts practical advice, thoughtful guidance, and unwavering encouragement to others who find themselves in similar battles. With every page turned, readers will uncover the profound power of resilience, the enduring significance of faith, and the transformative impact of embracing a fitness regimen while adhering to medical advice.

"Victorious Steps: Triumph over Diabetes through Faith and Fitness" is an empowering testament to the indomitable spirit of the human soul. It serves as a reminder that with unwavering faith, determination, and a commitment to physical well-being, triumph over adversity is not only possible but within reach.

Embark on an incredible journey alongside Brighton, where you'll find the resilience to triumph over diabetes and embrace a life filled with empowerment. As you delve into this book, be sure to pay close attention to invaluable tips provided throughout. Additionally, you'll discover a wealth of helpful information and resources waiting for you in the book's concluding chapters.

Chapter 1

My Lifestyle Life before Diabetes

My name is Brighton, and before the diagnosis of diabetes, my life was brimming with vitality, energy, and a carefree spirit, even though I wasn't engaging in regular exercise. I led a busy life, constantly on the go, embracing every opportunity that came my way. My days were filled with work, socializing, and indulging in my favourite hobbies. I had a boundless supply of energy that seemed to fuel my every endeavour. Each day was like a new adventure, and I lived it to the fullest. My mornings were a burst of vitality. Professionally, I was on an upward trajectory. I had a job I was passionate about, working long hours with a determination to excel. The challenges that came my way were seen as opportunities for growth, and I approached them with enthusiasm.

My evenings were often reserved for spending quality time with friends and family. Whether it was cosy gatherings at home, spontaneous outings, or lively parties, I cherished the connections I had with the people in my life. Laughter and shared moments were the currency of my social life. Above all, my carefree spirit defined my approach to life. I rarely worried about the future, choosing instead to embrace each day as it came. Life was an exciting journey, and I eagerly embarked on new adventures, often with a sense of childlike wonder. Little did I know that a storm was brewing within my body, silently threatening to disrupt the life I held so dear.

Diabetes, a condition that would soon become a significant part of my life, was silently taking root. The eventual diagnosis of diabetes was a sudden and unexpected turning point. It was as if the vibrant colours of my life were momentarily dimmed. I had to come to terms with the fact that I needed to make significant changes to my lifestyle, including adopting a careful approach to my diet, incorporating regular exercise, and monitoring my blood sugar levels.

In those days, I was blissfully unaware of the existence and significance of diabetes. Although my mother had been diagnosed with the condition in 2001, I didn't explore much into understanding its complexities. It was just a word, a part of her life that seemed distant and detached from my own. I had witnessed her managing the condition, but the impact it could have on my own life had not yet become a reality. I remember my mother's daily routine of checking her blood sugar levels, taking her medication, and carefully monitoring her diet. She would occasionally mention how important it was to maintain control over her blood sugar, but I never truly grasped the gravity of what she was going through. To me, it was just another part of her daily routine, like brushing her teeth or making breakfast. It wasn't until years later that I began to understand the impact of diabetes on my mother's life and the lives of millions of others who live with this condition.

Looking back, I realize how naïve I was. Diabetes isn't just a routine; it's a lifelong battle that requires constant vigilance and careful management. It's a condition that can have serious consequences if not properly controlled. But in those days, I was too preoccupied with my own concerns and

14

interests to fully appreciate the significance of my mother's struggle. Little did I know that diabetes would soon become a defining factor in my own life, reshaping my priorities and teaching me invaluable lessons about health and resilience.

Unbeknownst to me, there was a strong history of diabetes in both my mother's and father's sides of the family. It was a genetic thread woven into the fabric of my existence, silently waiting to manifest itself in my own journey. My uncle and aunt had battled with diabetes, but their struggles seemed distant and disconnected from my own life. On my mother's side, the prevalence of diabetes was a shadowy secret that only revealed itself when health complications arose. I would hear vague mentions of distant relatives who had struggled with their health, but the true nature of their battle was never fully explained. Similarly, on my father's side, the spectre of diabetes loomed large. Though it had not been openly discussed, I noticed patterns of dietary restrictions and health-conscious habits. Relatives would carefully watch their sugar intake and engage in regular exercise, but the underlying reason for these behaviours remained unspoken. It was as if diabetes had become an unacknowledged family tradition, passed down from one generation to the next. It wasn't until my mother herself was diagnosed with diabetes that the pieces of the puzzle began to fall into place. Suddenly, the family tree seemed to bear the weight of this genetic legacy, and I realized that diabetes was not just a random occurrence but a part of our shared genetic heritage. I never took the time to truly grasp the implications of their experiences or educate myself about the condition that could potentially shape my future.

In hindsight, I wish I had been more aware and understanding of diabetes when my mother was first diagnosed. Perhaps then, I could have offered her even more support and made her journey a little easier. But I've learned that it's never too late to educate oneself and become an advocate for a cause that affects someone you love. Diabetes may have once been a distant concept to me, but now it's a part of my life, and I'm determined to do my part in raising awareness and supporting those who live with it every day. Understanding the extent of diabetes in my family's history was both eye-opening and a cause for concern. It highlighted the importance of genetics in shaping our health and underscored the need for proactive measures to mitigate the risk. It also became a catalyst for my personal journey to learn more about diabetes, its causes, prevention, and management. In retrospect, the discovery of diabetes in my family history was a wake-up call, prompting me to take control of my health and encouraging open conversations about this condition among family members. It underscored the importance of knowing one's genetic predispositions and actively working to break the cycle of inherited health challenges. Through education, awareness, and proactive steps, we can strive to rewrite our family's health narrative for the better.

Going back to my pre-diagnosis days, as I reflect upon those times, I can't help but recognize the innocence and naivety that painted my perspective on life. It was an era when I lived in a bubble of invincibility, believing that youth and good fortune would be my armour against any potential health concerns. Little did I know that I was unwittingly laying the groundwork for my eventual diabetes diagnosis through a set of habits that, in hindsight, proved to be contributing factors.

As I reflect upon those days, I understand the innocence and naivety that coloured my perspective. I developed a set of habits that, in hindsight, were contributing factors to my eventual diagnosis.

In my younger days, health concerns seemed remote and abstract. I saw myself as someone who could eat anything without repercussions, who could go through life with minimal exercise, and who didn't need to pay much attention to what I consumed. My eating habits were far from ideal. Fast food and processed meals became staples in my diet due to my hectic schedule and the convenience they offered. I gave little thought to the importance of a balanced diet or the impact of my food choices on my long-term health. Healthy eating seemed like an abstract concept reserved for those who had the luxury of time and resources. My diet consisted of convenient fast food, sugary snacks, and oversized portions, and I rarely thought twice about it. Physical activity was sporadic at best, as the demands of a busy life often took precedence over regular exercise.

Pre-diagnosis experiences and Warning signs!

In my youthful ignorance, I dismissed the warnings about maintaining a balanced lifestyle. I shrugged off the importance of a well-balanced diet, regular check-ups, and exercise. After all, I felt invincible, shielded by my youthful energy and apparent good health. The consequences of my choices seemed distant and inconsequential. Exercise, too, took a backseat in my life. While I occasionally engaged in walks or embarked on weekend hikes, consistent physical activity was not a priority. I was sedentary for the most part, relying on bursts of energy and the demands of daily life to

17

keep me going. I failed to recognize the vital role that exercise plays in maintaining overall health and preventing the onset of chronic conditions.

Exercise? It felt like something from a bygone era, a distant memory of my younger, more energetic self. Back then, physical activity was a part of my daily routine, something I didn't have to think twice about. But as the years went by and the demands of work, family, and other responsibilities piled up, I slowly drifted into a sedentary existence. It was a complacency that had crept into my life, one that allowed these demands to consume my time and energy without question. Physical activity plays a crucial role in maintaining overall health and preventing the onset of diabetes. However, before my diagnosis, my exercise habits were less than optimal. I was leading a predominantly sedentary lifestyle, spending long hours sitting at a desk in my office. I would spend loads of hours watching football, especially my favourite team Manchester United. Definitely, lack of physical activity can contribute to weight gain and insulin resistance, and in my case this was obvious.

The consequence of this complacency was evident every morning when I dragged myself out of bed. Instead of feeling refreshed and ready to tackle the day, I felt like I was dragging a heavy anchor behind me. I woke up every morning feeling tired and sluggish, and a sense of dread would wash over me as I contemplated the day ahead. My sedentary lifestyle had taken a firm grip on my body, and I couldn't ignore the toll it was exacting any longer. I knew deep down that I was not doing enough to take care of myself, and it was starting to show. My energy levels were perpetually low, and I struggled to find the motivation to face the challenges ahead. It seemed like a relentless cycle of fatigue and frustration, and I knew it couldn't go on like this.

When it came to eating, I had unwittingly developed some truly terrible habits over the years. Fast food and processed snacks had insidiously become staples in my diet, and I had grown alarmingly accustomed to their convenience. Sugary drinks and indulgent desserts were regular treats, and I often found myself reaching for them without a second thought, disregarding the potential consequences they might have on my health. It was a routine of indulgence, instant gratification, and, ultimately, self-neglect.

The concept of balanced meals and portion control was virtually foreign to me. I would routinely skip breakfast, grabbing whatever was quickest on my way out the door. Lunches and dinners were often hasty affairs, centred around processed, high-calorie convenience foods that required minimal effort to prepare. Vegetables and fruits were rarely on the menu, and if they were, they were relegated to the role of garnish rather than the main event.

I had developed a sweet tooth that knew no bounds. Desserts, be they decadent cakes, creamy ice creams, or tempting pastries, were my Achilles' heel. I would indulge in them frequently, not considering the impact on my waistline or, more importantly, my overall health.

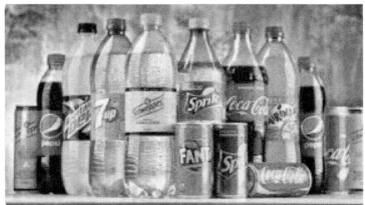

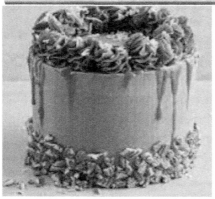

Sugary drinks were a constant companion throughout the day. Sodas, energy drinks, and even fruit juices filled my beverage choices, providing an instant sugar rush that I had grown reliant upon. Water, a fundamental element of a healthy diet, was often overlooked in favour of these sugary alternatives.

In essence, I had fallen into a trap of convenience and instant gratification. I chose what was easy and readily available, without ever stopping to consider the long-term effects on my well-being. It was a lifestyle that prioritized momentary pleasure over my health, and it had consequences that were beginning to catch up with me.

Stress became an ever-present shadow in my life, looming larger and darker as the years passed. The relentless pressure to meet deadlines at work and the challenges of managing personal relationships weighed heavily on my shoulders, casting a cloud of anxiety and tension over my existence. Little did I know that this chronic stress would play a pivotal role in the onset of my battle with diabetes, impacting both my mental and physical health in profound ways.

As the demands of my daily life escalated, I found myself seeking solace in all the wrong places. Instead of actively seeking out healthy ways to cope with the mounting stress, I turned to unhealthy vices as a means of temporary escape. The connection between my stress and the development of diabetes was not immediately apparent to me. It was as if my body had been silently registering the toll of chronic stress over time, and it finally began to send distress signals that couldn't be ignored. Excessive snacking, often on sugary and comfort foods, was my way of self-soothing, but it came with a hefty price. The uncontrolled consumption of unhealthy snacks had contributed to weight gain, high blood sugar levels, and other risk factors associated with diabetes.

Looking back, I can see that stress was not the sole cause of my diabetes, but it was a significant contributor. My journey with this condition has taught me the importance of addressing stress in healthier ways, not only to manage diabetes but also to lead a more fulfilling and balanced life. Stress will always be a part of life, but how we choose to cope with it can make all the difference in our long-term health and happiness.

Unbeknown to me, my body had been sending subtle warning signs that I chose to ignore. However, as the years passed, those seemingly inconsequential choices began to catch up with me. The occasional fatigue I felt turned into a persistent lack of energy. My sudden cravings for sugary snacks escalated into uncontrollable urges. My waistline expanded, and my weight crept up without warning. I attributed these changes to stress, a busy life, or the natural course of aging, never once suspecting that I was laying the groundwork for a health crisis. Fatigue became a constant companion, especially in the afternoons when a wave of exhaustion would wash over me. My insatiable thirst became a daily struggle, prompting me to reach for sugary drinks in an attempt to quench it. Frequent trips to the restroom became routine, as if my body was desperately trying to rid itself of an unseen burden.

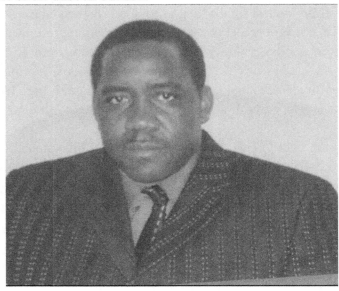

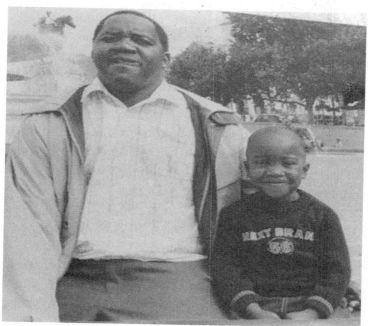

Pre- Diabetes : Brighton in 2007 Unaware of the "Storm brewing" inside me.

I was feeling constantly fatigued, experiencing frequent headaches, and struggling with unexplained weight gain. Over time, these signs grew more pronounced, and I couldn't ignore them any longer. Something was clearly amiss with my health, but fear and denial initially held me captive.

One of the earliest signs that something was wrong was excessive thirst. I found myself constantly reaching for a glass of water, my thirst unquenchable. It was as if my body was trying to tell me that something was not right, but I brushed it off, attributing it to the weather or other factors.

Frequent trips to the toilet, both during the day and at night, also became a routine part of my life. It felt as though I couldn't go more than a short while without needing to relieve myself. This constant urge to urinate was another warning sign that I chose to ignore, chalking it up to drinking more water.

My appetite began to fluctuate wildly. I would go from moments of instant hunger, where I felt like I could devour anything in sight, to times when I had no interest in food at all. These erratic shifts in appetite left me puzzled and unable to establish a consistent eating routine.

Sweating profusely became another daily occurrence. It seemed as though my body's temperature regulation was out of whack, and I was frequently drenched in sweat even when the weather wasn't particularly warm. This was yet another symptom that I couldn't explain or attribute to any specific cause.

Numbness and tingling sensations began to creep into my extremities, particularly my hands and feet. These sensations were unsettling and often left me feeling anxious. It was as if my body was trying to communicate that something was seriously wrong, but I was hesitant to confront the reality of what might be happening.

Despite these mounting signs and symptoms, fear and denial held me back from seeking medical attention. I convinced myself that I was simply going through a rough patch and that these issues would resolve on their own. Little did I know that these were the early indicators of a significant health challenge—my eventual diagnosis of diabetes.

Innocently unaware of the storm brewing within, I continued to live my life with a sense of invincibility. I carried on with my fast-paced lifestyle, giving little thought to the potential consequences of my choices. I indulged in fast food and processed meals, often relying on them for their convenience amidst my hectic schedules. I never stopped to consider the impact of a balanced diet on my long-term well-being.

Little did I know that this chapter of my life—the chapter before diabetes—would serve as a stark contrast to the journey that lay ahead. It was a chapter characterized by innocence and naivety, a time when I took my health for granted. The storm within was building momentum, and soon, it would demand my attention in ways I could never have anticipated. In retrospect, I'm grateful for the wake-up call that my diabetes diagnosis provided. It forced me to confront my unhealthy eating habits and make necessary changes to prioritize my health. While the path to healthier eating was not always easy, it ultimately became a source of empowerment and a vital component of managing my condition and regaining control over my well-being.

Looking back, I realize that acknowledging these signs and seeking medical help earlier could have led to an earlier diagnosis and a more proactive approach to managing my health. Diabetes was lurking in the shadows, and these warning signs were its way of urging me to take action.

In the upcoming chapters, I will delve into the defining moments of my journey with diabetes—the diagnosis, the initial resistance, the battles, and ultimately, the triumphs. These chapters will be a candid exploration of the highs and lows, the triumphs and tribulations that have shaped my experience since that pivotal diagnosis. Through my story, I hope to shed light on the challenges faced by those living with diabetes and inspire others to take control of their own health and well-being. My path would be arduous, but it would also be filled with valuable lessons, unwavering determination, and the realization that even in the face of adversity, a life of victory and empowerment is possible.

Tips!

Diabetes is a chronic medical condition that affects how your body processes glucose, which is a type of sugar and a primary source of energy for your cells. The hormone insulin, produced by the pancreas, plays a crucial role in regulating glucose levels in the bloodstream. Diabetes occurs when there is a problem with insulin production, action, or both, leading to elevated blood sugar levels.

There are several types of diabetes, with the two most common being:

Type 1 Diabetes: This is an autoimmune condition where the immune system mistakenly attacks and destroys the insulin-producing beta cells in the pancreas. People with type 1 diabetes must take insulin regularly through injections or an insulin pump to manage their blood sugar levels. It often develops in childhood or adolescence but can occur at any age.

Type 2 Diabetes: This is the most common form of diabetes and usually develops in adulthood, although it is becoming more prevalent in children and teenagers. In type 2 diabetes, the body becomes resistant to the effects of insulin, and the pancreas may not produce enough insulin to maintain normal blood sugar levels. Lifestyle factors, genetics, and obesity can contribute to the development of type 2 diabetes. Management typically involves lifestyle changes, oral medications, and, in some cases, insulin therapy.

Other less common types of diabetes include gestational diabetes (which occurs during pregnancy) and various forms of monogenic and secondary diabetes, which are typically associated with specific genetic or medical conditions.

The key symptoms of diabetes include:
- Frequent urination
- Increased thirst and hunger
- Unexplained weight loss
- Fatigue
- Blurred vision
- Slow-healing wounds or frequent infections

Uncontrolled diabetes can lead to serious health complications, including heart disease, stroke, kidney disease, nerve damage (neuropathy), vision problems, and foot problems that may result in amputation. However, with proper management, which includes monitoring blood sugar levels, a healthy diet, regular exercise, and medications as needed, people with diabetes can lead healthy and fulfilling lives while minimizing the risk of complications.

Chapter 2

Diagnosis and initial Reaction

Prior to that defining moment, I had been experiencing a series of symptoms that had gradually escalated in intensity. Frequent trips to the restroom and an unquenchable thirst had become a daily occurrence. I found myself guzzling down glasses of water, only to be left with an insatiable desire for more. It was as if my body was desperately trying to eliminate an unseen burden, and I was helplessly caught in the midst of it.

The pivotal moment arrived on September 1st, 2007. As the clock neared 8 pm that evening, a compelling urge led me to take action. I decided to conduct a blood sugar level test, using the glucometer I had purchased for my mother. The outcome was nothing short of staggering—32 mmol/L—a stark and undeniable indication that something was profoundly amiss. Panic and fear surged through my veins as I grasped the gravity of the situation. It was abundantly clear that immediate medical attention was an imperative necessity.

With a sense of urgency, I called 999, and an ambulance was dispatched to rush me to a local hospital in London. The journey was filled with a mix of emotions—fear, uncertainty, and a glimmer of hope that medical professionals would be able to provide answers and solutions. It was a pivotal moment that marked the beginning of my journey toward understanding and managing diabetes.

Upon arriving at the hospital, I was met by a team of healthcare professionals who swiftly attended to my needs. Blood pressure readings revealed another concerning aspect of my health—the numbers were elevated, indicating hypertension. The simultaneous presence of diabetes and high blood pressure added a layer of complexity to my diagnosis, but it also underscored the urgency with which I needed to address my health.

Initial reactions and emotional struggles

The voice of the doctor still echoes in my mind, his words etched into my memory with vivid clarity. "Brighton, you have diabetes, and you are hypertensive." The day of my diabetes diagnosis was a turning point that I will never forget. It was a moment that seemed to halt the world around me, and in its stillness, I found myself grappling with a whirlwind of emotions—fear, disbelief, and uncertainty. I will recount the details of that fateful day, the conversations with healthcare professionals, and the daunting reality of a life-altering condition that had suddenly become mine to navigate. It was a moment that brought the reality crashing down upon me, shattering any illusions of invincibility I had held onto. Hearing those words hit me like a ton of bricks. I never thought I would be at risk for a chronic illness at this stage of my life. It was a wake-up call, a stark reminder that I needed to make drastic changes to my lifestyle. It wasn't until the fateful day of my diabetes diagnosis that the bubble of invincibility burst. I was confronted with the consequences of my past habits, and it was a wake-up call I couldn't ignore. My initial shock and disbelief gradually gave way to a profound sense of regret for not taking better care of my health earlier on. Looking back, I realize that my pre-diagnosis days were marked by a sense of complacency, an illusion of immortality that allowed me to ignore the warning signs. But I've since learned that health is a fragile gift, one that requires conscious effort and responsibility.

I couldn't help but feel a sense of disbelief. How could this happen to me? I had seen my mother struggle with diabetes, witnessed the challenges it presented in her life, and yet somehow, I had convinced myself that I would be exempt from such a fate. The truth was, diabetes had a stronghold in my family history, with both my mother and paternal side having been diagnosed with the condition. It was a stark reminder of the importance of understanding and addressing genetic predispositions. I couldn't escape the realization that I was now part of a lineage of individuals who had fought this battle before me. It was a wake-up call, forcing me to confront the reality of my own vulnerability. I had been aware of this risk, but in my youthful naivety, I brushed it off as something that wouldn't touch my own life. Diabetes, coupled with hypertension, seemed like an insurmountable mountain to climb. The combination of these two conditions only amplified the challenges I would face in managing my health. It was a double blow, a one-two punch that left me reeling with uncertainty. But it wasn't just the diagnosis that defined my journey; it was also the initial resistance. I'll share the stories of denial, of grappling with the enormity of the changes I needed to make, and of the moments when I questioned whether I had the strength to face this challenge head-on. It was a period marked by self-doubt and the weight of adjusting to a new normal.

31

In that very instant, my world turned upside down. Waves of emotions crashed over me like a tidal wave—fear, disbelief, and a deep sense of loss. It felt as though I had been handed a life sentence, a burden I was ill-prepared to bear. Questions swirled relentlessly in my mind, each one a heavy burden, begging for answers that felt increasingly elusive. The day I received my diabetes diagnosis was a life-altering moment that left me grappling with an overwhelming sense of uncertainty and doubt. It wasn't just the medical facts and dietary adjustments that consumed my thoughts; it was the existential questions, the ones that pierced the very core of my being.

"How did this happen to me?" was the initial query that echoed through my thoughts. I combed through my memories, searching for clues or warning signs that I had missed. I couldn't comprehend how this condition had stealthily taken root in my body, seemingly out of nowhere. It was a feeling of betrayal by my own physical form, and I yearned for a clear explanation that could bring me some semblance of understanding.

"What does this mean for my future?" was another question that loomed large. I envisioned a future coloured by medications, insulin injections, and constant vigilance over my blood sugar levels. It was a stark departure from the life I had known, and I couldn't help but wonder how it would impact my aspirations, my relationships, and my overall quality of life.

And then there was the haunting question, one that echoed in the deepest recesses of my mind: "Can I overcome this?" Doubt gnawed at my confidence, and I grappled with the fear of failure. Could I truly manage this condition, make the necessary lifestyle changes, and emerge victorious in my battle with diabetes?

But perhaps the most profound and perplexing question of all was the one that touched upon matters of faith: "Why did God allow this to happen to me?" I questioned the very foundations of my faith, wondering if this diagnosis was a test of my belief or a punishment for some perceived failing. Had I been lacking in faith, and was this the consequence?

In the midst of these questions and doubts, I sought solace in my faith. It was a complex journey of rediscovering the strength of my beliefs and reconciling them with the challenges before me. I turned to prayer for guidance, searching for answers and seeking the peace that only faith could provide. It was in these moments of reflection and contemplation that I began to find a semblance of clarity.

I began to see my journey with diabetes as an opportunity to grow spiritually, to strengthen my faith, and to find meaning in the challenges I faced. It was a reminder that adversity can be a catalyst for personal growth and a testament to the human spirit's ability to overcome.

In the end, my questions persisted, but they no longer held the same power to paralyze me with fear and doubt. Instead, they became a catalyst for self-discovery and a source of motivation to confront my diagnosis with unwavering determination. My faith, once shaken, emerged stronger than ever, reminding me that even in the face of life's most profound questions, there is room for faith to flourish.

The initial shock of the diagnosis gave way to a rollercoaster of emotions. I felt anger, directed both inwardly and outwardly. I was angry at myself for neglecting my health, for ignoring the warning signs, and for allowing diabetes to take hold of my body. I was angry at the world—for being so unjust, for burdening me with this relentless condition. I found myself seething with anger at myself, first and foremost. It was a deeply internalized fury, a resentment that I couldn't easily shake off. I was furious with myself for neglecting my health for so long, for allowing the warning signs to go unnoticed or wilfully ignored. I berated myself for the poor choices I had made, the unhealthy lifestyle I had led, and the complacency that had allowed diabetes to take hold of my body. Each guilty thought was like a heavy stone, weighing me down with regret and self-recrimination. But my anger didn't stop with self-directed blame. It extended outward, like a wildfire consuming everything in its path. I felt anger at the world, at the universe itself, for being so seemingly unjust. It felt like an unfair burden, an unrelenting sentence, one that I didn't deserve. I questioned why this had to happen to me, why I had to contend with a condition that seemed so relentless and unforgiving. I felt a profound sense of injustice, as if life had thrown me an incredibly cruel curveball.

Fear gripped me tightly, its icy fingers wrapping around my heart. I feared the unknown, the complications that could arise, and the limitations that diabetes might impose on my life. Thoughts of the future filled me with anxiety—would I be able to manage this disease? Would it hinder my dreams, my ambitions? But in that moment, as the doctor's words sank in, a fire ignited within me—a determination to rise above my circumstances and find a way to conquer this new reality.

In the midst of these emotions, a profound sense of loss washed over me. I mourned the life I once knew, the carefree days before diabetes cast its shadow upon me. I mourned the freedom to eat without worry, the spontaneity that had been replaced by meticulous planning. It felt as though a part of me had been taken away, forever altered by this unwelcome intruder. I was admitted in hospital for a week. I had a lot of reflection whilst in a London hospital. Lots of thoughts raced my mind! A lot of them I must say!

The realization that I was diabetic fuelled a newfound determination within me. I refused to let diabetes dictate my life; I refuse to be another statistic. I knew I needed to prioritize exercise, even if it means starting small and gradually building up my stamina. I was going to make an effort to incorporate physical activity into my daily routine, whether it was going for walks, taking up a sport, or joining a gym. Moreover, this newfound awareness served as a powerful motivator to make positive lifestyle changes not only for myself but also for future generations. I recognized the significance of a healthier lifestyle, regular check-ups, and heightened vigilance regarding the warning signs of diabetes. It was not just about breaking the cycle but also about ensuring that my own children and grandchildren would inherit a legacy of health and well-being rather than a legacy of silent, familial diabetes.

Revamping my eating habits was going to be another essential step. I was going to educate myself about proper nutrition and make conscious choices that support my health.

Fresh fruits and vegetables, lean proteins, and whole grains was going to become the foundation of my meals. I was going learn to cook nutritious meals at home, reducing my dependence on processed foods and dining out.

Stress management was also going to become a priority. I thought of exploring different techniques such as meditation, and deep breathing exercises to find inner peace and alleviate the pressures of daily life. Seeking support from loved ones and possibly joining support groups to provide the encouragement and guidance I needed to stay on track. Over time, as I grappled with this emotional storm, I began to recognize that anger was a natural response to a life-altering diagnosis like diabetes. It was a manifestation of the grief and upheaval that comes with such a profound change in one's life. It was a reaction to the loss of the life I had known before, the freedom I had taken for granted, and the innocence I had lost.

Acknowledging and addressing this anger became an essential part of my journey with diabetes. It forced me to confront my emotions, to seek support from loved ones and healthcare professionals, and to channel that anger into productive avenues. It pushed me to advocate for myself, to learn more about my condition, and to make the necessary changes to manage it effectively.

Tips!
When you receive a diabetes diagnosis, it's natural to experience a range of emotions and reactions as you come to terms with this new aspect of your life.

Shock and Disbelief: Initially, you might feel shocked and find it hard to believe that you have diabetes. It's common to question how this could happen to you.

Fear and Anxiety: As the reality sets in, fear and anxiety about the future may take hold. Worries about complications, managing your condition, and needing medications or insulin can be overwhelming. Uncertainty about what lies ahead can be scary.

Sadness and Grief: You might start to feel sadness and a sense of loss. It's not unusual to grieve for the lifestyle you had before the diagnosis, especially if it involved enjoying certain foods or activities without restrictions.

Anger and Frustration: Some people experience anger and frustration. You might direct these emotions at yourself, wondering why you didn't prevent the condition, or you may feel that life is unfair and ask, "Why me?"

Confusion and Overwhelm: Understanding how to manage diabetes can be confusing, and the sheer volume of information may overwhelm you. Dietary changes, medication routines, and the need to monitor your blood sugar levels may seem daunting at first.

Motivation to Change: On the flip side, a diabetes diagnosis can serve as a powerful motivator for positive change. You may become determined to adopt a healthier lifestyle, including dietary improvements, regular exercise, and quitting unhealthy habits.

Seeking Information and Support: Realizing the importance of knowledge and support, you actively seek information. You reach out to healthcare providers, diabetes educators, support groups, and reliable online sources to educate yourself about diabetes management.

Social Support: The presence of supportive family and friends can make a significant difference. Their emotional encouragement and willingness to assist you with practical matters can provide comfort during this challenging time.

Acceptance: Over time, you begin to accept your diabetes diagnosis. You realize that it's a part of your life but not your entire identity. Acceptance involves acknowledging the condition and making a commitment to manage it effectively.

Empowerment: Some individuals view their diagnosis as an opportunity to take control of their health. You might become proactive in managing your diabetes, attending regular check-ups, and making informed decisions about your care.

Remember that your emotional journey is unique, and it's okay to experience these reactions at your own pace. Over time, as you become more familiar with diabetes management and gain confidence in your ability to handle it, your emotions may evolve, and you can take proactive steps toward living a healthy and fulfilling life with diabetes. Seeking guidance and connecting with a supportive community can greatly aid in your diabetes journey.

Education

The days following my diagnosis were a whirlwind of medical appointments, tests, and a crash course in diabetes management. I found myself confined within the walls of a London hospital, where a team of dedicated healthcare professionals worked tirelessly to stabilize my condition and equip me with the knowledge, I needed to navigate life with diabetes.

It wasn't until my diabetes diagnosis that I was forced to confront the gravity of my dietary choices. I had to re-evaluate my entire approach to food and nutrition. It was a daunting challenge, but it was also a wake-up call I sorely needed.

I began to educate myself about the importance of a balanced diet and the role it plays in managing diabetes. I learned to read food labels, understand the glycemic index, and make healthier choices. Fruits and vegetables started to make regular appearances on my plate, and I began to appreciate the variety and flavors they brought to my meals.

I also had to break free from my sugar addiction. It was a difficult journey filled with cravings and temptations, but with time, I learned to savor the sweetness of naturally occurring sugars in fruits and the occasional, carefully chosen indulgence. Sugary drinks were replaced with water and herbal teas, allowing me to stay hydrated without the detrimental effects of excessive sugar consumption.

The transformation in my eating habits was not only a necessity for managing diabetes but also a profound shift in my perspective on food. I came to realize that food should nourish and sustain, not just provide fleeting pleasure. It was a journey of self-discovery and self-care, one that required patience and determination.

During that week-long stay, the hospital indeed became my temporary home, and the medical staff, my trusted guides in this new and unfamiliar territory. They embarked on a meticulous journey to unravel the complexities of my health, conducting a battery of tests that each played a crucial role in painting a comprehensive picture of my condition. The process was overwhelming, but I understood that these tests were absolutely essential in piecing together the puzzle of my health.

Blood Glucose Monitoring: This was one of the first tests performed. The medical team needed to gauge my blood sugar levels over time to confirm the diabetes diagnosis. Regular blood glucose checks provided a baseline for understanding how my body was processing sugar.

Hemoglobin A1c Test: This test provided a longer-term view of my blood sugar control. It measured the average blood glucose levels over the past two to three months, offering insight into how well I had been managing my condition even before the diagnosis.

Fasting Blood Sugar Test: This test involved measuring my blood sugar after an overnight fast. It helped determine whether my body was able to maintain healthy blood sugar levels when I wasn't eating.

Oral Glucose Tolerance Test (OGTT): In this test, I was asked to drink a sugary solution, and my blood sugar levels were monitored at intervals afterward. It helped assess how my body processed sugar and whether there were any abnormalities.

Lipid Profile: This test examined my cholesterol levels, including LDL (bad cholesterol) and HDL (good cholesterol). Diabetes can increase the risk of heart disease, so monitoring cholesterol was essential.

Kidney Function Tests: Diabetes can affect kidney function over time, so tests to assess kidney health were a crucial part of the treatment. This often involved measuring creatinine levels and glomerular filtration rate (GFR).

Liver Function Tests: These tests were conducted to check the health of my liver, as diabetes could impact liver function. They assessed markers like alanine aminotransferase (ALT) and aspartate aminotransferase (AST).

HbA1c: Hemoglobin A1c, or glycated hemoglobin, was another important marker for assessing long-term blood sugar control. It provided insights into how well my diabetes management was working over a span of several months.

Blood Pressure Monitoring: High blood pressure often accompanies diabetes and can further complicate health issues. Regular blood pressure checks were essential to evaluate and manage this aspect of my health.

Eye Exams: Diabetes can affect vision, so I underwent comprehensive eye exams to monitor for any signs of diabetic retinopathy or other eye-related complications.

Foot Exams: Given that diabetes can lead to nerve damage and poor circulation in the feet, regular foot exams were conducted to catch any issues early and prevent complications.

Each of these tests served as a vital piece of the diagnostic and management puzzle, helping the medical team tailor a comprehensive treatment plan for my specific needs. While the battery of tests was undoubtedly overwhelming, they were essential steps in my journey towards understanding and managing my condition effectively.

As the days passed during my hospital stay, I found myself increasingly immersed in a world of diabetes education. It was an enlightening and necessary process, and the healthcare team played an indispensable role in guiding me through this transformative phase of my life. They patiently and compassionately explained the intricacies of my diagnosis, emphasizing that I had been diagnosed with type 2 diabetes, a condition that would now shape my daily life.

One of the most profound lessons I received was about the underlying mechanisms of type 2 diabetes. The medical professionals took the time to demystify this complex condition, breaking it down into digestible pieces of information. They explained that type 2 diabetes is characterized by insulin resistance, a situation in which the body's cells do not respond effectively to insulin, a hormone responsible for regulating blood sugar levels. This newfound knowledge allowed me to grasp the root cause of my condition, empowering me with a deeper understanding of what was happening inside my body.

Understanding the significance of blood sugar regulation became a cornerstone of my diabetes education. The healthcare team stressed its paramount importance and explained that keeping blood sugar levels within a healthy range was crucial for preventing complications and maintaining overall well-being. They taught me about the role of carbohydrates in raising blood sugar and how various factors, such as diet, exercise, and medication, could influence these levels.

I learned about the importance of glycemic control, which involved managing the intake of carbohydrates, monitoring blood sugar levels, and making informed decisions about meals and snacks. This knowledge gave me a sense of agency over my condition, as I realized that my daily choices could significantly impact my health.

Additionally, the healthcare team delved into the various tools and techniques I could use to monitor my blood sugar levels effectively. I became familiar with glucose meters, which allowed me to check my blood sugar at home, and I was taught how to interpret the results. This monitoring process would become an integral part of my daily routine, enabling me to track my progress and make adjustments as needed.

While the medical interventions were crucial, it was the lessons about life with diabetes that truly resonated with me. The healthcare professionals patiently walked me through the dos and don'ts of diabetes management. They educated me about the importance of monitoring my blood sugar levels regularly, adhering to medication regimens, and making necessary dietary adjustments.

I learned that managing diabetes was not simply about taking medications—it was about adopting a holistic approach to my health. I discovered the significance of maintaining a balanced diet, incorporating regular physical activity into my daily routine, and prioritizing self-care. The healthcare team emphasized that diabetes was a lifelong condition, but one that could be managed effectively with the right tools and mindset.

Their teachings extended beyond the physical aspects of diabetes. They addressed the emotional and psychological challenges that often accompanied the diagnosis. They emphasized the importance of self-compassion, resilience, and seeking support from loved ones and diabetes support groups. They assured me that I was not alone in this journey and that there were resources available to help me navigate the emotional ups and downs that may arise.

Beyond the technical aspects of diabetes management, the healthcare team also emphasized the importance of a holistic approach to my well-being. They encouraged me to adopt a healthy lifestyle that included a balanced diet, regular physical activity, stress management, and adequate sleep. These lifestyle changes were not just recommendations; they were essential components of my diabetes management plan, designed to promote better health and reduce the impact of the condition on my life.

In retrospect, this intensive diabetes education was transformative. It empowered me with knowledge, dispelled fears, and gave me the tools to take control of my health. It marked the beginning of my journey towards a life that was not defined by diabetes but rather guided by an informed and proactive approach to well-being. It was a profound chapter in my life, one that would ultimately shape my perspective on health and resilience in the face of adversity.

The treatment plan that the healthcare team put in place during my hospital stay was nothing short of comprehensive. They recognized the urgency of addressing my immediate needs and ensuring that I left the hospital with a solid foundation for managing my newly diagnosed type 2 diabetes. As a result, they introduced me to a combination of medications and therapies designed to bring my blood sugar levels under control and stabilize my condition.

One of the key components of my treatment plan was insulin therapy. Insulin injections were administered to help regulate my blood sugar levels promptly. The medical team carefully determined the appropriate dosage and schedule, ensuring that my insulin regimen was tailored to my specific needs. This immediate intervention was crucial in getting my blood sugar levels under control and preventing potential complications.

In addition to insulin, I was prescribed metformin tablets, a medication commonly used to treat type 2 diabetes. Metformin works by improving the body's response to insulin, reducing the amount of sugar produced by the liver, and enhancing the uptake of sugar by the cells. It played a pivotal role in managing my blood sugar levels and improving my overall insulin sensitivity.

Another medication introduced as part of my treatment plan was a sitagliptin tablet. Sitagliptin belongs to a class of drugs known as dipeptidyl peptidase-4 (DPP-4) inhibitors. It works by increasing the levels of certain hormones in the body that stimulate the pancreas to produce more insulin and decrease the amount of sugar produced by the liver. This medication complemented the other therapies in helping maintain stable blood sugar levels.

The combination of insulin, metformin, and sitagliptin aimed to address my immediate and long-term needs, with the goal of stabilizing my condition. The healthcare team closely monitored my response to these medications, making adjustments as necessary to achieve optimal blood sugar control.

However, the treatment plan extended beyond medication. The healthcare professionals also provided extensive education on dietary management, encouraging me to adopt a balanced diet that included controlled carbohydrate intake. They emphasized the importance of regular physical activity and stress management in managing blood sugar levels effectively. I was equipped with the knowledge and tools necessary for ongoing self-care and management of my condition.

As I prepared to leave the hospital, I did so with a newfound sense of empowerment. The comprehensive treatment plan had not only addressed my immediate health concerns but also set me on a path toward long-term well-being. Armed with medications, knowledge, and a supportive healthcare team, I was ready to face the challenges of life with type 2 diabetes and embark on a journey of self-care and resilience.

As the days drew to a close and I prepared to leave the hospital, I felt a mixture of emotions—gratitude for the care I had received, apprehension about the road ahead, and a newfound determination to take charge of my health. I knew that my life had changed irrevocably, but I also understood that this diagnosis did not define me. It was an opportunity for growth, for self-discovery, and for embracing a new way of living.

Tips on food!

Breakfast ideas when you have diabetes.

Diabetes won't stop you from enjoying your food, but knowing some simple hacks and swaps will help you choose healthier options and make planning your meals a little easier. These ideas may not look much different from what you eat already, and your favourite recipes and meals can usually be adapted to be healthier without you noticing too much difference.

Here are some healthy breakfast ideas to choose from:

- a bowl of wholegrain cereal with milk
- two slices of wholegrain toast with olive oil-based spread
- a pot of natural unsweetened yogurt and fruit
- two slices of avocado with a hardboiled egg.

Switch from white toast to wholegrain versions like seeded batch bread, multi-seed, granary, soya and linseed. These are better for your diabetes and digestive health. They're more filling, too.

If you're making rotis and chapattis, use wholewheat flour.

- Instead of jam try mashed banana.
- Other healthy choices are low-fat cheese, cottage cheese with a couple of fresh chopped dates, or nut butter (make sure the one you buy doesn't have any additions like sugar or palm oil) and chopped banana.
- Try to limit the amount of oil when cooking. Cook with unsaturated vegetable oils, such as sunflower, olive or rapeseed, instead of butter or ghee.
- Add extra fruit and veg to bump up your fibre intake wherever you can.
- Add berries, dried fruit or half a banana to your cereal, or grilled tomatoes to eggs on toast.

Breakfast drinks

Even pure fruit juices and smoothies contain free sugars, and it's easy to consume a lot in one go. It's better to eat whole fruit and veg, but if you do have a juice or smoothie, limit the portion to 150ml once a day and try making your own.

If you're buying coffee on the go, be on the lookout for added syrups and purees, which contain a lot of free sugars. If you're not sure, ask the server to tell you what ingredients are used in your favourite drink.

Lunch ideas when you have diabetes

Here are some healthy lunch ideas to choose from:

- a chicken or tuna salad sandwich.

- a small pasta salad.

- soup with or without a wholegrain roll.

- a piece of salmon or tuna steak and salad.

Think about having a piece of fruit or a pot of natural unsweetened yogurt afterwards too.

Dinner ideas when you have diabetes

- Here are some healthy dinner ideas to choose from:
- lasagne and salad
- roast chicken and vegetables, with or without potatoes
- beef stir-fry and vegetables, with or without brown rice

chicken tortillas and salad

salmon and vegetables, with or without noodles

curry with chickpeas and brown rice

Get more dinner recipes – you can search by type of meal and ingredient.

Can I eat fruit?

Yes, whole fruit is good for everyone and if you have diabetes, it's no different. You shouldn't avoid them because they're sugary. Fruits do contain sugar, but it's natural sugar. The sugar in whole fruit is different to the added sugar in things like chocolate, biscuits and cakes or other free sugar found in fruit juices and smoothies.

Other things to avoid are foods labelled 'diabetic' or 'suitable for diabetics', and eating too much red and processed meat or highly processed carbs like white bread. Cutting down on these means you're reducing your risk of certain cancers and heart diseases.

Vegetables

Load up! Vegetables are among the healthiest forms of carbs. You'll get lots of fiber. And unless you add salt or fat, they have very little of both.

Best Choices

- Fresh veggies -- raw, lightly steamed, roasted, or grilled
- Plain frozen vegetables lightly steamed.
- Greens such as kale, spinach, and arugula.
- Tabouli and other types of nutrient-rich salads,
- Low-sodium or unsalted canned vegetables.

Chapter 3

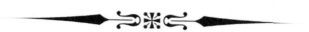

Battling the Effects of Diabetes
Physical and emotional toll on your well-being

Living with diabetes presents an array of challenges that extend far beyond the initial diagnosis. It is a relentless battle against a condition that seeks to disrupt every aspect of my life—physically, emotionally, and mentally. In this chapter, I will delve into the multifaceted effects of diabetes and how they have shaped my journey.

The physical toll of diabetes is undeniable. Fluctuating blood sugar levels became a constant concern, demanding constant vigilance and careful monitoring. High blood sugar left me feeling lethargic, mentally foggy, and physically drained. Low blood sugar episodes were equally challenging, with their dizzying spells, trembling limbs, and an overwhelming sense of vulnerability. Simple tasks that once came easily suddenly required an extra effort. The weight of fatigue pressed upon me, making even the most mundane activities feel like an uphill battle. I longed for the boundless energy of my pre-diabetic days, but I knew that managing my blood sugar levels was essential for my long-term health and well-being.

But it wasn't just the immediate effects of blood sugar fluctuations that impacted me. Over time, diabetes took its toll on various parts of my body. It brought about a dizzying array of symptoms that left me feeling weak, shaky, and disoriented. Trembling limbs and a rapid heartbeat became unwelcome companions during these episodes. The fear of losing control and experiencing a severe hypoglycemic event lingered at the back of my mind, urging me to take swift action to raise my blood sugar levels. I carried snacks with me at all times, prepared to combat the sudden drops in glucose levels that could occur unpredictably. The importance of regular check-ups and screenings became apparent as I faced potential complications such as nerve damage, kidney problems, and cardiovascular issues. Each new challenge served as a reminder of the stakes involved, propelling me to take proactive steps towards managing my condition.

I quickly learned that diabetes was more than just a physical condition—it had a profound impact on my emotional well-being as well. The daily fluctuations and the fear of potential complications weighed heavily on my mind. It was not uncommon to experience moments of overwhelm and vulnerability, questioning whether I had the strength to face the challenges that lay ahead. Emotionally, diabetes placed a heavy burden on my well-being. The constant worry and anxiety surrounding my health became a constant companion. The fear of long-term complications loomed over me, leading to moments of despair and vulnerability. It was a delicate balance between acknowledging the gravity of the situation and finding the strength to persevere. It demanded a heightened sense of self-awareness, constantly monitoring how I felt and checking my blood sugar levels regularly. It was a reminder that I needed to be proactive in managing my health, with no room for complacency. However, there were moments of frustration and feelings of helplessness when despite my best efforts, my blood sugar levels veered off course.

Experiences with managing blood sugar levels, medications, and other treatments

Managing blood sugar levels became a daily ritual, a delicate dance of timing, dosages, and self-awareness. It involved meticulous monitoring, carbohydrate counting, and adjusting insulin or oral medications as needed. Adhering to a proper diet became paramount, with a focus on balanced meals, portion control, and understanding the impact of different foods on my blood sugar levels.

In my journey of managing diabetes, medications and treatments have been pivotal in maintaining stability and optimizing my overall well-being. From the very moment of my diagnosis, I understood the importance of adhering to the prescribed regimen, knowing that these medications would play a significant role in controlling my blood sugar levels and mitigating the risks associated with diabetes.

One of the key components of my treatment plan has been insulin injections. Insulin became an essential part of my daily routine, requiring careful administration and monitoring. Learning to inject myself with insulin initially felt daunting, but with guidance from healthcare professionals and the support of my loved ones, I soon developed the confidence and proficiency to handle this aspect of my diabetes management. It became a ritual— checking my blood sugar levels, calculating the appropriate insulin dosage, and administering the injection at the recommended times throughout the day.

Adhering to the prescribed medication regimen required discipline and responsibility. It became a non-negotiable part of my daily routine, ingrained into the fabric of my life. I developed strategies to ensure that I never missed a dose, whether it meant setting alarms or carrying my medications with me wherever I went. I understood that consistency was crucial in achieving optimal blood sugar control and mitigating the risks associated with diabetes.

Beyond medications, I also embraced other treatments that complemented my diabetes management. Regular visits to my healthcare team became a priority, allowing for ongoing monitoring of my health and adjustments to my treatment plan as necessary. These appointments served as a platform for open and honest discussions about my progress, concerns, and any challenges I faced. With their guidance and expertise, we worked together to fine-tune my treatment plan, ensuring that it aligned with my unique needs and goals.

Support Groups
Beyond the conventional treatments, I explored complementary therapies and lifestyle changes to further support my diabetes management. Navigating the challenges of diabetes can be overwhelming, but finding support through diabetes support groups has been instrumental in my journey towards better management and overall well-being. These groups provide a safe and understanding space where individuals with diabetes come together to share experiences, exchange advice, and offer each other emotional support.

Joining a diabetes support group was a turning point for me. It allowed me to connect with others who were facing similar struggles and triumphs, creating a sense of solidarity and understanding that I had longed for. In these groups, I discovered a wealth of knowledge, wisdom, and first-hand experiences that helped me navigate the complexities of diabetes.

One of the most significant benefits of diabetes support groups has been the exchange of practical information. Members freely share tips and techniques they have learned through their own journeys, ranging from strategies to manage blood sugar levels to advice on medication regimens and dietary choices. This shared knowledge has expanded my understanding of diabetes management and empowered me to make informed decisions about my health.

The emotional support I received from these groups has been invaluable. Diabetes can sometimes feel isolating, as the day-to-day challenges and constant vigilance can take a toll on mental and emotional well-being. However, through support groups, I found a network of compassionate individuals who truly understood the emotional impact of living with diabetes. We shared our frustrations, fears, and successes, offering empathy, encouragement, and a listening ear. The sense of camaraderie and understanding that emerged from these connections helped alleviate feelings of loneliness and provided a renewed sense of hope.

Additionally, support groups often invite guest speakers, experts, and healthcare professionals who provide valuable insights and address specific topics related to diabetes management. These sessions offer opportunities for education, enabling members to stay informed about the latest research, treatment options, and self-care practices. The knowledge gained from these presentations has helped me make more informed decisions about my own diabetes management and enhanced my overall well-being.

Beyond the regular support group meetings, online communities have also played a vital role in my diabetes journey. Online platforms provide a convenient space for individuals from different geographical locations to connect and share their experiences. These communities offer continuous support, allowing members to seek advice, share resources, and find encouragement whenever needed. The 24/7 accessibility of online support groups has been particularly beneficial during times of urgency or when seeking immediate assistance or reassurance.

Through diabetes support groups, I have formed lasting friendships with individuals who understand the intricacies of living with diabetes. We celebrate each other's victories, provide a shoulder to lean on during challenging times, and inspire one another to persevere. The support and camaraderie I have experienced within these groups have given me strength, motivation, and the confidence to face the daily demands of managing diabetes.

Through the trials and tribulations of my journey with diabetes, I have come to understand that it is not merely a physical condition; it is an all-encompassing battle that demands resilience, adaptability, and an unwavering commitment to self-care. Diabetes is a relentless adversary that affects every facet of life, from daily routines to long-term plans. It has tested my resolve, challenged my preconceptions, and forced me to confront my vulnerabilities. However, in the midst of these challenges, I have also discovered that diabetes can be a catalyst for personal growth and empowerment.

The challenges of diabetes have been many, from the meticulous management of blood sugar levels to the ever-present spectre of potential complications. The need for constant vigilance and discipline can be emotionally taxing, and there have been moments of frustration, fear, and doubt. Yet, in facing these challenges head-on, I have unearthed reservoirs of strength and determination I never knew I possessed.

Resilience has become a core trait in my battle with diabetes. It's the ability to bounce back from setbacks, to persevere in the face of adversity, and to adapt to the ever-changing landscape of this condition. It's not just about enduring; it's about thriving despite the odds. The daily management of diabetes may be relentless, but it has cultivated a spirit of resilience within me, reminding me that I am stronger than I ever imagined.

Adaptability has also played a pivotal role in my journey. Diabetes demands flexibility in lifestyle, diet, and daily routines. It requires the ability to adjust and find creative solutions to unexpected challenges. It has taught me to be nimble in the face of change and to embrace the process of trial and error as I navigate the intricacies of my condition.

Perhaps the most profound aspect of this journey has been the discovery of self-empowerment. Diabetes forced me to take ownership of my health and well-being. It prompted me to educate myself, to seek out the support of healthcare professionals, and to make informed decisions about my lifestyle and treatment. In doing so, I have reclaimed a sense of control over my life that I once thought had been lost.

Diabetes has also instilled a deep appreciation for the importance of self-care. It is a daily reminder that prioritizing my health is not a luxury but a necessity. It has taught me to value the gift of good health and to recognize that self-care is an act of self-love.

As I reflect on my journey, I am reminded that adversity has the power to shape us in profound ways. Diabetes is not a battle I would have chosen, but it is one that has enriched my life in unexpected ways. It has honed my resilience, nurtured my adaptability, and empowered me to take charge of my health. It has shown me that even in the face of formidable challenges, a life of fulfilment and purpose is not only possible but achievable.

So, as I continue to navigate the complexities of diabetes, I do so with a heart full of gratitude for the lessons it has bestowed upon me. It is a reminder that the human spirit has an incredible capacity for growth and that, even in the midst of adversity, we can emerge stronger, wiser, and more empowered than ever before.

Tips!

Battling the effects of diabetes involves managing your condition effectively to prevent or minimize complications. Here are some important tips to help you in this battle:

Regular Medical Check-Ups: Schedule regular appointments with your healthcare team, including your primary care physician, endocrinologist, and other specialists. These check-ups will help monitor your overall health and diabetes management.

Blood Sugar Monitoring: Monitor your blood sugar levels regularly as recommended by your healthcare provider. Keeping your blood sugar within target ranges can reduce the risk of complications.

Medication Adherence: Take your prescribed medications as directed. If you have concerns about your medication, discuss them with your doctor before making any changes.

Healthy Eating: Follow a balanced and diabetes-friendly meal plan. Pay attention to portion sizes, choose complex carbohydrates, prioritize vegetables and lean proteins, and limit sugary and high-fat foods.

Physical Activity: Incorporate regular physical activity into your routine. Aim for at least 150 minutes of moderate-intensity aerobic exercise per week, along with strength training exercises at least two days a week.

Weight Management: Achieve and maintain a healthy weight. Even a modest weight loss can have a significant impact on blood sugar control.

Smoking Cessation: If you smoke, make a plan to quit. Smoking can exacerbate diabetes-related complications.

Blood Pressure Control: Monitor and manage your blood pressure. High blood pressure can increase the risk of heart disease and kidney problems.

Cholesterol Management: Keep your cholesterol levels in check. High cholesterol is a risk factor for heart disease, especially for people with diabetes.

Foot Care: Inspect your feet daily for any cuts, sores, or blisters. Proper foot care is essential to prevent complications like diabetic neuropathy and foot ulcers.

Eye Exams: Schedule regular eye exams with an eye specialist to detect and treat diabetic retinopathy, which can lead to vision problems.

Kidney Health: Maintain kidney health by managing your blood pressure and blood sugar, and getting regular kidney function tests.

Oral Health: Practice good oral hygiene to prevent gum disease, which can affect blood sugar control.

Stress Management: Find healthy ways to manage stress, such as through relaxation techniques, meditation, or hobbies you enjoy.

Support System: Lean on your support system, including family, friends, and support groups. Sharing your challenges and victories can be emotionally beneficial.

Education: Continuously educate yourself about diabetes and its management. Understanding your condition empowers you to make informed decisions.

Emergency Preparedness: Have a plan for diabetes management during emergencies or natural disasters. Ensure you have an emergency kit with essential supplies.

Vaccinations: Stay up-to-date on vaccinations, including the flu and pneumonia vaccines, as people with diabetes are more susceptible to infections.

Remember that managing diabetes is a lifelong journey, and it's essential to take a proactive and holistic approach to minimize its effects and complications. Work closely with your healthcare team, stay informed, and make healthy lifestyle choices to maintain the best possible health while living with diabetes.

In the forthcoming chapters, I will delve into the depths of my relapse phase, examining the reasons behind it, the detrimental effects it had on my physical and mental well-being, and the transformative impact of the wake-up call from my doctor. I will share the moments of struggle and self-discovery, the steps I took to rebuild my life, and the lessons I learned along the way. Through this chapter of my journey, I hope to inspire others who may find themselves in a similar relapse, reminding them that it is never too late to reclaim their health and rewrite their story of triumph over diabetes.

Chapter 4

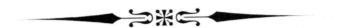

Massive Relapse!

Resistance to following professional advice and the consequences.

Accepting my diagnosis was not an easy feat. It required me to confront my fears, acknowledge my vulnerabilities, and let go of the notion that I was somehow immune to the challenges that millions of others faced daily. It was a humbling experience—one that taught me the importance of self-reflection and the need to take ownership of my health.

As days turned into weeks and months, I continued to challenge myself, reaching milestones I once deemed unreachable. Yet, life is a tapestry of unforeseen twists and turns, and in 2009, I found myself caught in a downward spiral—a massive relapse. I began to neglect my diabetes management, and inevitably, I faced the repercussions of my actions.

In the midst of grappling with the harsh reality of my diabetes diagnosis, an unexpected and defiant spirit began to stir within me. It was a tumultuous blend of emotions— pride, denial, and an overpowering desire to regain control over my life—that fueled my resistance to the professional guidance I had received. I convinced myself that I possessed superior knowledge, that I could manage my diabetes according to my own terms. This path was strewn with misconceptions, misguided beliefs, and a multitude of reasons that bolstered my resistance to acknowledging my diagnosis.

As I reflect on that period of my life, I must admit that complacency slowly seeped into my mindset. Over time, I began to take my progress for granted, convinced that I had conquered the condition. I veered off the strict routes I had set for myself, both in terms of exercise and diet. My once carefully planned meals became laden with excessive carbohydrates, and I indulged in a wide array of unhealthy food choices. The discipline and dedication that had once defined my diabetes management slipped away, and I found myself drifting further from the path of optimal health.

One of the primary reasons for my resistance was a deep-seated belief that divine intervention alone would heal me. I clung to the hope that, through faith and prayer, I could overcome this condition without the need for medical intervention. It was a testament to my unwavering trust in a higher power, a belief that sometimes led me to question whether seeking medical treatment was a sign of weak faith.

Denial played a significant role as well. I found myself questioning the accuracy of the diagnosis, almost as if by rejecting it, I could make it untrue. Diabetes was a formidable adversary, and acknowledging its presence felt like admitting defeat. I told myself that the tests must have been mistaken, that there had been some error, and that I didn't truly have this condition.

Pride was another driving force behind my resistance. I didn't want to be labelled as someone with a chronic illness. The idea of being dependent on medications or needing to make significant lifestyle changes clashed with my self-perception as a strong and independent individual. It was a battle of ego, a desire to prove to myself and others that I could handle this on my own.

I also fell victim to the misconception that diabetes was a condition that only affected those who were overweight or lived unhealthy lifestyles. I believed that my relatively healthy habits and physical appearance exempted me from this diagnosis. This misguided notion led me to downplay the seriousness of the condition and question why it had chosen me.

Furthermore, the fear of change played a role in my resistance. Adhering to a new diet, incorporating regular exercise, and managing medications seemed overwhelming. I was resistant to altering my daily routines and sacrificing the comforts of my old lifestyle. The idea of facing the unknown and adapting to a new way of life was daunting.

I disregarded the importance of regular blood sugar monitoring, convinced that I could rely solely on how I felt to gauge my body's needs. I dismissed the prescribed medications, convinced that they were unnecessary. And I stubbornly clung to my old habits, refusing to acknowledge the need for dietary changes and exercise.

Neglecting my doctor's appointments became a regular occurrence. The routine check-ups, which were essential in monitoring my blood sugar levels and ensuring the effectiveness of my treatment plan, fell by the wayside. I convinced myself that I knew best that I could manage my diabetes without external guidance. Little did I know that these decisions would have far-reaching consequences. However, these unhealthy food choices came at a cost. Excessive carbohydrate intake caused my blood sugar levels to spike, leading to erratic fluctuations that were difficult to control. The stability I had worked so hard to achieve slipped through my fingers as I lost sight of the importance of mindful eating and balanced nutrition.

Simultaneously, my exercise routine took a backseat. The consistent physical activity that had been an integral part of my diabetes management plan dwindled to a mere afterthought. I neglected my regular workouts, often making excuses or prioritizing other activities over exercise. The once-thriving commitment to fitness and its positive impact on my blood sugar control faded away, leaving a void that was quickly filled with sedentary habits.

As the discipline and dedication waned, I found myself drifting further from the path of optimal health. The detrimental effects of my relapse began to manifest physically, mentally, and emotionally. Physically, the weight I had diligently shed started to pile back on. The extra pounds put strain on my body, exacerbating the challenges I faced in managing my blood sugar levels and leading to a decline in overall energy and well-being. The effects of my relapse were devastating. Physically, I began to balloon once again, undoing all the progress I had achieved in weight loss. The pounds piled on, and the strain on my body became more pronounced. The extra weight took a toll on my energy levels, mobility, and overall well-being.

But as days turned into weeks, and weeks into months, the consequences of my resistance became painfully clear. Fluctuating blood sugar levels became my constant companion, leaving me drained and irritable. I experienced the consequences of neglecting my health—fatigue, blurred vision, and a host of other unsettling symptoms that served as reminders of the price I was paying.

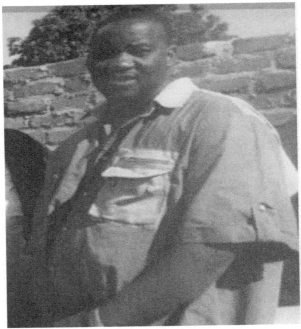

REPLASING

Yet, it was not only the physical effects that took a toll on me. The emotional and mental impact of my relapse was equally profound. Guilt, frustration, and a sense of failure enveloped me as I realized the magnitude of my complacency. The habits and routines that had once empowered me now felt distant and unattainable. I found myself caught in a cycle of self-doubt, questioning whether

I would ever regain control of my health. Mentally, I trapped in a downward spiral of despair and hopelessness. The realization of my relapse and its implications on my health left me feeling overwhelmed and filled with self-doubt. Emotionally, I found myself caught in a vicious cycle. The apprehension of my relapse and the consequences of my neglect gnawed at me, fuelling self-doubt, guilt, and a sense of failure.

The consequences of my relapse were significant. I watched in dismay as the numbers on my glucose meter spiralled out of control. Elevated blood sugar levels brought with them a cascade of symptoms—constant thirst that could never be quenched, the urgency to urinate frequently, and an unrelenting fatigue that seemed to weigh me down with each passing day. It was a stark reminder that neglecting my diabetes management came at a steep price.

It was during this period of reckoning that I realized the futility of my resistance. I came face to face with the harsh reality that I couldn't fight diabetes with stubbornness alone. I needed to swallow my pride, accept the professional advice, and make the necessary changes to regain control of my health.

In the midst of this despair, I sought out a doctor's guidance, hoping for a glimmer of hope amidst the darkness. The encounter with my doctor was a wake-up call like no other. With a grave expression, he looked me in the eyes and spoke words that shook me to my core. "Brighton, unfortunately, you are going to die and leave your family if you don't change." The weight of those words hit me with a force I had never experienced before. It was a stark reminder of the severity of my relapse and the consequences of neglecting my diabetes management.

Facing the consequences of my neglect was a harsh wake-up call. It was a reminder that diabetes, while manageable, was a condition that required continuous diligence and commitment. Neglecting my health had dire consequences not only on my physical well-being but also on my overall quality of life.

However, it was also a humbling experience that served as a reminder of the resilience that had carried me through previous challenges. Just as I had once overcome the initial shock of my diagnosis, I knew that I had the strength to regain control of my health and steer myself back on the path of self-care.

The relapse of 2009 was a pivotal moment in my journey with diabetes. It taught me that managing this condition was not a linear progression but a continuous effort that required vigilance and adaptability. It was a lesson in humility and the importance of seeking support during difficult times.

As I reflect on this period of relapse, I am reminded that setbacks are a part of life, but they do not define us. The true measure of resilience lies in our ability to acknowledge our missteps, learn from them, and move forward with renewed determination. My journey with diabetes had its share of ups and downs, and this relapse was just one chapter in a larger narrative of resilience, growth, and self-discovery.

In hindsight, I can see that my resistance to accepting my diabetes diagnosis was a complex and emotionally charged response. It was born out of a mixture of faith, denial, pride, misconceptions, and fear. However, as time passed and I gained a deeper understanding of the condition, I began to recognize the importance of embracing the professional advice and guidance that had been offered to me. It was a journey of transformation, one that required me to set aside my resistance and open myself to the possibilities of living a fulfilling life despite diabetes.

Tips!

Relapses in diabetes management can be challenging, but they are not uncommon. If you've experienced a relapse or are concerned about the possibility, here are some tips to help you get back on track:

Self-Compassion: Understand that relapses happen to many individuals managing chronic conditions like diabetes. Be compassionate with yourself and avoid self-blame.

Reflect on Triggers: Identify what triggered the relapse. Was it stress, a major life change, lack of motivation, or a change in routine? Understanding the trigger can help you address it.

Consult a Healthcare Professional: Reach out to your healthcare team, including your doctor, diabetes educator, and dietitian. They can provide guidance, adjustments to your treatment plan, and support.

Set Realistic Goals: Start with achievable goals. Don't overwhelm yourself with drastic changes. Small, sustainable steps are often more effective.

Monitor Blood Sugar: Regularly check your blood sugar levels to understand the impact of the relapse on your health. It can also help motivate you to make positive changes.

Revisit Your Diabetes Plan: Review your diabetes management plan with your healthcare team. Ensure it's tailored to your current needs and lifestyle.

Meal Planning: Reevaluate your meal plan and focus on balanced, nutritious choices. Consider consulting a dietitian for guidance.

Physical Activity: Gradually reintroduce physical activity into your routine. Start with light exercises and gradually increase intensity.

Medication Adherence: If you're on medication, ensure you're taking it as prescribed. Set reminders if necessary.

Support System: Lean on your support network, including family and friends, for encouragement and assistance in your diabetes management journey.

Seek Behavioural Support: Consider talking to a therapist or counsellor who specializes in behavior change to address any underlying issues contributing to relapses.

Join a Diabetes Support Group: Participating in a support group can provide motivation, share experiences, and offer practical tips.

Track Your Progress: Keep a journal to record your meals, physical activity, and blood sugar levels. Tracking your progress can be motivating.

Celebrate Achievements: Acknowledge and celebrate your successes, no matter how small. Positive reinforcement can help maintain motivation.

Stay Informed: Continuously educate yourself about diabetes management. The more you understand, the better equipped you'll be to make informed choices.

Stay Hydrated: Proper hydration is essential. Drinking enough water can help regulate blood sugar levels.

Sleep: Prioritize quality sleep as it plays a significant role in blood sugar control and overall well-being.

Plan for Cravings: Acknowledge that cravings may arise, and have healthy snacks readily available to manage them.

Remember that managing diabetes is a lifelong journey, and setbacks can happen. What's important is your commitment to getting back on track and taking steps to improve your health and well-being. Don't hesitate to seek professional help and rely on your support system to assist you in overcoming relapses.

In the subsequent chapters, I will share the transformative journey that unfolded as I embraced the wisdom of healthcare professionals, relinquished resistance, and embarked on a path of self-care and empowerment. Through my experiences, I hope to inspire others to overcome their own resistance, accept the guidance available to them, and embark on a journey of healing and triumph. I will share the highs and lows, the victories and setbacks, and the moments of revelation that have shaped my fight against diabetes. I will share the transformative moments, the lessons learned, and the strategies I have employed to reclaim control of my health and lead a fulfilling life despite the challenges that diabetes presents. Through my story, I hope to inspire others facing similar battles to find their own strength, embrace faith, and adopt a fitness regime that can lead them to a life of victory over this relentless condition.

Chapter 5

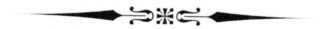

Running Towards Wellness: From Couch to Marathon

The wake-up call of that relapse in 2009 was a jolt to my complacency like no other. It was a stark reminder of the consequences of neglecting my diabetes management, and it ignited a fire within me—a fire that rekindled the determination and resilience I had once possessed. In the face of adversity, I realized that I had a choice to make: to succumb to my circumstances or to rise above them. It was a pivotal moment of self-reflection and resolve, and I made a solemn vow to reclaim my health, to fight back against this relentless condition with every ounce of strength I had left.

The realization that I had let myself slip into complacency was humbling and humbling and served as a catalyst for change. I recognized that I could not afford to take my health for granted, and I could not allow diabetes to hold me hostage. I had conquered challenges before, and I was determined to do so again.

With unwavering determination, I set out on a journey of self-renewal and transformation. It began with a commitment to re-establishing the habits that had once empowered me. Reflecting on my journey towards wellness, one particular date stands out with profound significance: July 27, 2011. On that pivotal day, I made a deliberate and life-altering decision to seize control of my health and initiate a change. The words of my doctor echoed in my ears, acting as an unwavering reminder of the critical importance of prioritizing my well-being. This moment served as a clarion call, a stark realization that I had reached a juncture where action was not just advisable but imperative. It was my wake-up call, propelling me into a new phase of my life, one in which my health took precedence.

The decision to incorporate regular exercise into my life was undeniably clear. I recognized that physical activity was a cornerstone of effective diabetes management and overall well-being. However, the question that lingered was: where do I begin? The prospect of embarking on a fitness journey felt both exhilarating and intimidating. I knew I needed to take that first step, and after careful consideration, running emerged as the ideal avenue to commence this transformative path.

Running held a unique allure for me. It symbolized freedom, empowerment, and the boundless potential of the human body. It embodied simplicity—a practice that involved putting one foot in front of the other, each stride symbolizing progress, and each step resonating with determination. Running felt like a metaphor for my broader journey to reclaim my health and well-being, promising not just physical exertion but mental and emotional rejuvenation. It seemed like the perfect way to challenge myself physically, engage in cardiovascular exercise, and harness the power of my own body. I knew that running had the potential to transform not only my physical fitness but also my mental and emotional well-being. However, the start of my running journey was far from easy. I can vividly recall the day I laced up my running shoes for the first time. Those shoes were not just footwear; they were instruments of transformation. With every lace secured, it felt as though I was cinching away the weight of complacency and self-doubt. The inaugural run was modest—a tentative jog rather than a full-fledged sprint—but it was an initiation, a critical initial step in the right direction.

I began by walking, slowly building up my endurance and preparing my body for the more intense challenge of jogging. As time went on, I felt a growing sense of readiness to progress from walking to jogging. It was a natural transition, fuelled by the desire to challenge myself and unlock the full potential of my physical capabilities. I started incorporating short jogging intervals into my walks, gradually increasing the duration and intensity. The key was consistency and gradual progression, allowing my body to adapt and grow stronger over time. Consistency became my guiding principle. Despite the cold weather in the UK, I never allowed it to deter me from my commitment to running. I laced up my shoes and hit the pavement, regardless of the elements. The more I ran, the more I discovered the transformative power of this form of exercise. Regular walks helped me to gradually build up my endurance and strengthening my body. Each day, I pushed myself a little further, determined to lay a solid foundation for my running endeavors. It took months of consistent effort before I felt ready to transition from walking to jogging. I vividly remember hitting the roads of London, determined to conquer each step and push myself further.

In those nascent stages, running was a formidable challenge. My body, accustomed to a sedentary lifestyle, protested against the newfound exertion, and my lungs gasped for breath. However, beneath the physical discomfort, I sensed positive changes unfolding within me. The rhythm of my breath, the pulsating beat of my heart, and the sensation of my muscles working in unison became tangible indicators of progress and vitality.

As I persisted in my running regimen, I discovered solace in the steady rhythm of my footsteps. Running evolved into a form of meditation, a sanctuary where I could escape the cacophony of the world and discover inner tranquility. The path ahead, while physically demanding, was mentally liberating—a space where I could introspect, set fresh goals, and chart the course for my future.

Running also served as a conduit for reconnecting with the natural world. I explored parks, trails, and scenic routes, immersing myself in the beauty of nature. Each run became an adventure—an opportunity to embrace the sights and sounds of the outdoors, a stark contrast to my previous sedentary existence.

Over time, my unwavering dedication to running yielded tangible results. My stamina improved, my weight began to stabilize, and, most significantly, my blood sugar levels became more manageable. It was a testament to the remarkable power of physical activity as a tool for diabetes management and overall well-being.

Yet, beyond the physical benefits, running transformed into a symbol of empowerment. It became a potent reminder that

I possessed the agency to make choices that would mould my health and my life. It exemplified that I could transcend the limitations of my condition and expand my horizons in pursuit of a healthier and more vibrant future.

Decision Day!

The decision to commence running on that pivotal day, July 27, 2011, marked a profound turning point in my journey towards wellness. It was a choice forged in resolute determination, fuelled by the urgency of my health, and grounded in the unwavering belief that transformation was attainable. Running became a transformative force that propelled me forward on the path to better health, instilling in me the unwavering conviction that, even in the face of adversity, I had the capacity to seize control of my health and embrace a life filled with vitality and purpose.

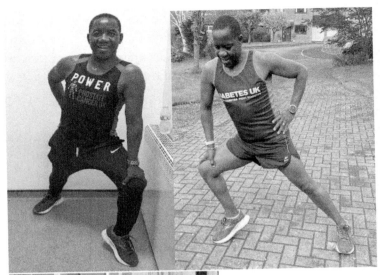

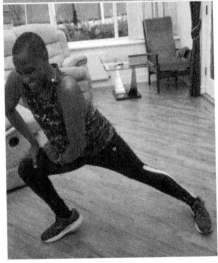

Brighton: Started to shrink again because of
exercising

To keep myself motivated and accountable, I set achievable goals along the way. I would challenge myself to jog a little longer or cover a slightly longer distance during each session. These small milestones provided a sense of accomplishment and fuelled my determination to push further. I also sought inspiration from other runners, reading books and articles about running journeys and following the achievements of renowned athletes. Their stories served as a reminder that with dedication and perseverance, I too could reach new heights. My running journey was marked by significant milestones and accomplishments. It's important to note that starting a running journey requires patience and self-compassion. It's a process of self-discovery, embracing both the triumphs and the challenges. It's about understanding that progress may come gradually, and setbacks may occur along the way. It's crucial to listen to your body, honouring its limits while also pushing beyond at you thought possible.

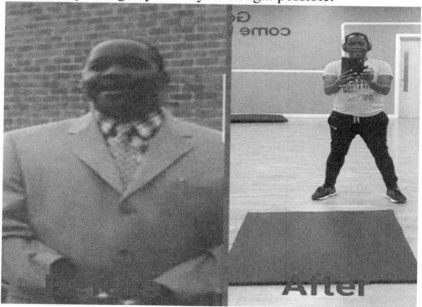

Edinburgh- Scotland Marathon (42.2 Km)

The transition from 10km runs to tackling the full marathon was a significant milestone in my running journey. It marked a moment of both excitement and apprehension as I prepared to push my physical and mental limits to new heights. It was during this time that I decided to participate in my first marathon, which took place in the beautiful city of Edinburgh, Scotland.

The anticipation leading up to the race was palpable. I had put in months of dedicated training, gradually building my endurance and preparing my body for the gruelling 42.2-kilometer challenge ahead. The nerves coursed through my veins as I joined the sea of runners, each one with their own goals and aspirations.

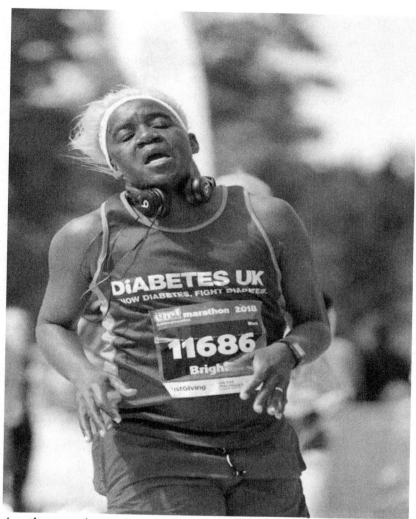

As the starting gun echoed through the air, a surge of adrenaline propelled me forward. The first few kilometres were a whirlwind of excitement, surrounded by fellow runners and the supportive cheers of spectators. I found myself settling into a rhythm, the rhythmic pounding of my footsteps reverberating in my ears.

The marathon route in Edinburgh was a true testament to the city's beauty and charm. It was a journey that allowed me to not only test my physical endurance but also to soak in the rich tapestry of this historic city. As I traversed the course, I found myself captivated by the breath-taking landscapes, enchanted by the winding streets steeped in history, and inspired by the iconic landmarks that graced the path.

The marathon route took us on a remarkable tour of Edinburgh's heart and soul. We wound our way through historic streets, where centuries of stories and memories seemed to linger in the very cobblestones beneath our feet. It was as if the past and present converged in those narrow lanes, and with each stride, I felt connected to the city's vibrant heritage.

One of the most exhilarating aspects of the route was the opportunity to pass by iconic landmarks. The sight of Edinburgh Castle perched atop its rocky fortress was awe-inspiring, a symbol of the city's resilience and grandeur. As I ran, I couldn't help but appreciate the juxtaposition of ancient architecture against the backdrop of a modern marathon, a testament to the enduring spirit of this remarkable place.

The views offered along the way were nothing short of spectacular. Edinburgh's natural beauty unfolded before my eyes as I made my way through the course. Whether it was the sweeping vistas of the Pentland Hills or the serene shores of the Firth of Forth, each panorama served as a reminder of the breath-taking landscapes that Scotland had to offer.

But what truly made the marathon memorable was the incredible atmosphere that enveloped the event. The camaraderie among the runners was palpable, a shared sense of purpose and determination that transcended words. We were all united by a common goal—to conquer the challenge set before us and to push our limits.

As the kilometres began to tick by during the marathon in Edinburgh, the full scope of the physical and mental challenges became increasingly apparent. Fatigue settled in, and doubts started to creep into my mind like persistent shadows. The weight of the distance ahead seemed daunting, and the voice of uncertainty whispered, "Can you really do this?"

However, in those critical moments, I reached deep within myself, drawing upon the wellspring of determination and resilience that had brought me to this point. It was not just the marathon I was running; it was a battle against my own limitations, a challenge I had willingly undertaken in my crusade against diabetes.

I reminded myself of the countless hours I had devoted to training, pounding the pavement in the early morning hours and pushing myself to the limits during late-night runs. Each step I took on that marathon course was a testament to the dedication and discipline I had cultivated over the months.

In those dark moments when doubt threatened to engulf me, I thought about the purpose that had driven me from the beginning. I was not merely running for personal glory or achievement; I was running to defeat diabetes, to show that this condition did not define me but that I was the one defining its limits. It was a mission that went beyond the marathon—it was a declaration of my determination to conquer adversity and take control of my health.

The thought of the countless individuals who faced similar struggles with diabetes spurred me on. I knew that my journey was not just about my own triumph; it was about inspiring others to take charge of their health and defy the odds. With each step, I carried the hopes and aspirations of those who were battling diabetes alongside me, and I refused to let any obstacles hinder my progress.

The marathon became a metaphor for the challenges of living with diabetes. It was a test of endurance, a battle against the odds, and a testament to the power of the human spirit. With every stride, I overcame not only physical fatigue but also the doubts that had once held me back.

The marathon in Edinburgh was not just a solitary endeavour; it was a collective experience, made all the more powerful by the support of the crowd and the camaraderie among the runners. The spectators who lined the streets played a pivotal role in fuelling my motivation and helping me push through the physical and mental barriers of the race.

As I ran, I could hear the cheers and applause of the spectators ringing in my ears. Their encouraging words and enthusiastic shouts became a lifeline during moments when my energy waned, and doubt threatened to creep in. Each "You've got this!" and "Keep going!" was like a shot of adrenaline, a reminder that I was not alone in this journey.

What made the experience even more poignant was the fact that I was running for a cause close to my heart—I was running to support Diabetes UK. Many of the spectators along the route were individuals who had a personal connection to diabetes, whether they were living with the condition themselves or supporting loved ones who were. Their cheers were not just for me but for everyone who had been touched by diabetes. We were all united by a common goal—to conquer the marathon and raise awareness about diabetes. In that shared pursuit, we became a community, bound together by our determination and our collective mission.

I vividly remember the Diabetes UK supporters who had come out to cheer me on. They wore shirts emblazoned with the organization's logo, and their energy was infectious. Their presence was a powerful reminder of the impact of the work we were doing to support those affected by diabetes and to fund research for a cure. As I ran past these dedicated supporters, their cheers took on a deeper meaning. It was not just about completing a marathon; it was about making a difference in the lives of individuals and families affected by diabetes. Their support was a reminder that our efforts were contributing to a brighter future for those living with the condition.

The marathon was a true testament to the power of community and the strength that comes from coming together to pursue a shared goal. In those challenging moments when fatigue threatened to overwhelm me, the collective support of the crowd and the shared determination of my fellow runners propelled me forward.

As I approached the final stretch, the emotions intensified. The finish line stood before me like a beacon of triumph, drawing me closer with every stride. With every ounce of energy, I had left, I summoned a surge of determination, sprinting towards the finish line with a mix of exhaustion and exhilaration.

Crossing the finish line of the Edinburgh marathon was a moment of pure, unadulterated elation. It was a culmination of months of hard work, dedication, and unwavering determination. As I crossed that threshold, a rush of emotions swept over me, leaving me nearly breathless with a profound sense of achievement.

Completing my first marathon was an accomplishment that, at one point in my life, I had considered utterly impossible. The weight of that achievement washed over me like a tidal wave, and it was accompanied by a surge of
could hardly capture.

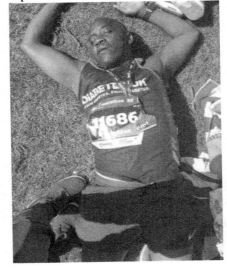

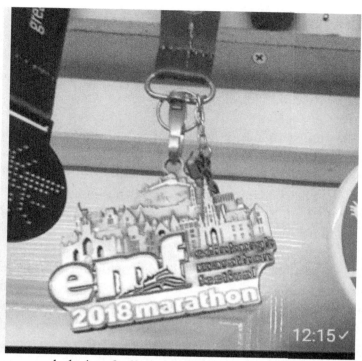

The overwhelming feeling that engulfed me at that moment was pride—pride in myself, pride in the progress I had made, and pride in my victory over diabetes. It was a testament to the power of perseverance, an affirmation that no challenge is insurmountable when met with unyielding determination.

My finishing time of 4 hours and 17 minutes exceeded my own expectations. It was a clear measure of the growth I had experienced throughout my running journey. It reminded me of the countless hours of training, the early mornings when I had laced up my running shoes in the dark, and the late nights when I had pushed myself to go just a little bit farther. It was a validation of the progress I had made, not only in terms of my physical fitness but also in my battle against diabetes.

Victory over diabetes was not just a personal triumph; it was a message to the world that this condition could be managed and conquered. My journey served as an example of what could be achieved when one takes control of their health and refuses to let a medical diagnosis define their destiny.

In the midst of the crowd's cheers and applause, I felt a profound sense of gratitude—for the support of my family, friends, and the Diabetes UK community; for the countless individuals who had inspired me on this journey; and for the strength that had carried me through every mile of that marathon.

As I stood at the finish line, I couldn't help but reflect on how far I had come since my diabetes diagnosis. Running had become more than just a physical activity; it had become a symbol of resilience, a source of empowerment, and a beacon of hope for all those who faced the challenges of diabetes.

My victory over diabetes was not the end of my journey; it was a milestone in an ongoing quest for wellness and advocacy. It was a reminder that, no matter the obstacles we face, we have the power within us to overcome, to achieve, and to inspire others along the way.

In conclusion, crossing the finish line of my first marathon was a moment of triumph that transcended the boundaries of a mere race. It was a victory over diabetes, a celebration of the strength of the human spirit, and a testament to the power of perseverance and determination. It was a reminder that, in the face of adversity, we can achieve greatness and inspire others to do the same.

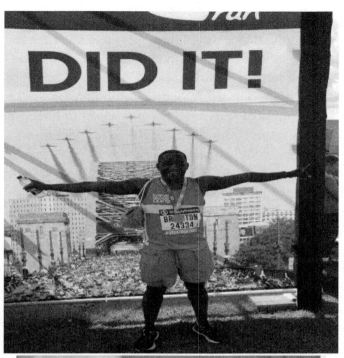

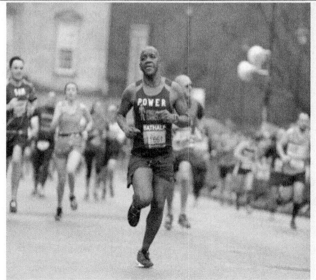

The marathon experience in Edinburgh ignited a fire within me, one that fuelled my passion for running and transformed it into an enduring obsession. I became a dedicated and enthusiastic runner, eagerly seeking out new challenges and races across the United Kingdom. Running became more than just a physical activity; it became a way of life, a source of inspiration, and a means to continue my victorious steps over diabetes. My running journey was not just about crossing finish lines; it was about breaking down stereotypes and challenging misconceptions about diabetes. It was about demonstrating that individuals living with diabetes could lead active, fulfilling lives and achieve remarkable feats. My mission was to empower others to take control of their health, one step at a time, and to let them know that they were not alone on this path. In summary, the marathon experience in Edinburgh marked the beginning of my passionate journey with running—a journey that transcended the physical act of running and became a powerful platform for diabetes advocacy and empowerment. From half marathons to races across the UK, I embraced each opportunity to run, inspire others, and prove that victory over diabetes was not only possible but also a source of strength and resilience.

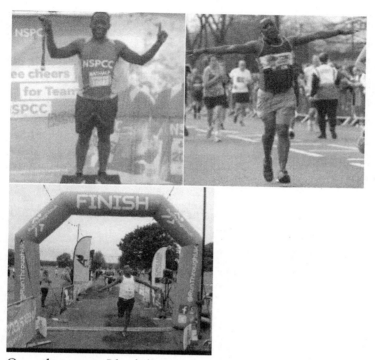

Over the years, I had the privilege of participating in over 20 half marathons. Each race was an opportunity to push myself to new limits, both physically and mentally. It was a chance to prove to myself and others that living with diabetes did not mean living with limitations—it meant breaking through barriers and reaching new heights.

The Manchester Full Marathon, the Great North Half Marathon, the Bath Half Marathon, Kingston Upon Thames, Stoke on Trent Half, Cheshire Half and countless other races became chapters in my ongoing journey of empowerment and advocacy. Each race was a platform for personal growth, a demonstration of my commitment to managing diabetes through an active lifestyle, and an opportunity to inspire others to take control of their own health.

I took pride in the fact that I was not just a runner but a symbol of triumph over adversity. Every step I took was a reminder that diabetes did not define me; rather, it was a challenge I had chosen to confront head-on. Through my running, I encouraged others facing similar battles with diabetes to do the same—to lace up their shoes, hit the pavement, and embrace the transformative power of physical activity.

Running has become a way for me to share my story and advocate for diabetes awareness. It was a tangible representation of the message that victory over diabetes was achievable. I was not running away from my condition; I was running with it, acknowledging its presence but refusing to let it hold me back.

I often found myself reflecting on how far I had come since that initial diagnosis. From a place of uncertainty and fear, I had emerged as a beacon of hope and empowerment. Each race, each victory, was a testament to the progress I had made, both in managing my diabetes and in inspiring others to do the same.

As the miles piled up in my running journey, I noticed a significant change occurring within me—I began to shed weight, both physically and metaphorically. Running emerged as a game changer in my life, a force that not only transformed my physical health but also had a profound impact on my mental and emotional well-being. The process of running, the rhythmic pounding of my feet on the pavement, and the steady flow of breath became more than just physical exercise; they became my source of empowerment and rejuvenation.

One of the most visible changes was the transformation of my physical body. The regularity and consistency of my running regimen led to a gradual reduction in weight. As the pounds melted away, I felt a newfound lightness in my step. Running was not just helping me manage my diabetes; it was reshaping my entire physique. The weight loss was a tangible manifestation of my commitment to well-being and a testament to the power of physical activity as a tool for transformation.

However, the impact of running extended far beyond the physical realm. It was a balm for my mental and emotional well-being. The act of running released a flood of endorphins, those natural feel-good chemicals, which enveloped me in a sense of euphoria and contentment. It was as if each run was a therapy session, washing away stress and anxiety, leaving me with a profound sense of calm and clarity.

The sense of accomplishment that followed every run became addictive. Setting a goal, whether it was a distance milestone or a time target, and then surpassing it filled me with a deep sense of pride and satisfaction. It reinforced the idea that I was not defined by my condition, but by my ability to overcome it through sheer determination and effort. Running became a metaphor for life itself—an endeavour in which challenges were meant to be conquered, not avoided.

Moreover, running became a way to escape from the noise and chaos of daily life. The solitude of the open road or the serenity of a park provided a precious respite from the pressures of work and personal responsibilities. It became a form of meditation, a time when I could clear my mind, reflect on my journey, and find solutions to life's challenges.

The discipline of running also spilled over into other aspects of my life. It instilled a sense of structure and routine that extended beyond the track or trail. I became more mindful of my dietary choices, recognizing that what I consumed directly impacted my performance as a runner and my overall health as an individual.

In summary, running was not merely an exercise; it was a catalyst for transformation. It reshaped my physical body, revitalized my mental and emotional well-being, and imbued me with a profound sense of accomplishment and self-belief. It was a reminder that even in the face of adversity, the human spirit has the power to triumph, one step at a time. Running was not just a means of managing my diabetes; it became a way of life, an embodiment of resilience, and a symbol of empowerment that would continue to shape my journey towards wellness.

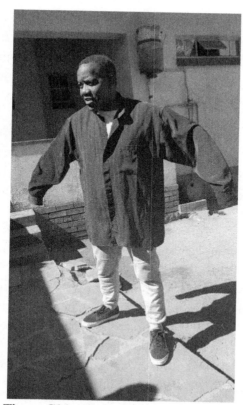

Testimony Time: Shirt that I used to wear when I was a "couch potato"

Even during the most challenging times, such as the onset of the COVID-19 pandemic, I remained resolute in my commitment to pursuing my passion for running, managing my diabetes, and maintaining my overall well-being. Adversity, rather than being a deterrent, became an opportunity for me to adapt, innovate, and find new ways to continue my fitness journey and inspire others along the way.

The pandemic brought with it a set of unprecedented challenges. Lockdowns, social distancing measures, and restrictions on outdoor activities disrupted the routines of many. However, I was determined not to let these obstacles deter me from my mission of running, advocating for diabetes awareness, and demonstrating the victorious steps that could be taken even in the face of adversity.

One of the first adjustments I made was to adapt my running routine to the new circumstances. With restrictions on outdoor activities in place, I turned to indoor running and home workouts. I discovered the power of technology and virtual races, connecting with fellow runners online and participating in virtual running events that brought the running community together, even when physically apart.

But my commitment to promoting fitness and diabetes management extended beyond my personal endeavors. I wanted to create a platform that would empower and motivate others to embrace physical activity, especially in the face of a global health crisis. Thus, I introduced an online initiative called "Will Power Sunday Roast."

"Will Power Sunday Roast" was a Facebook-based activity that I launched to reach out to a wider audience. Through this initiative, I shared a variety of exercises and workouts that people could easily do from the comfort of their own homes. The goal was to make fitness accessible and enjoyable for individuals of all fitness levels, regardless of their circumstances or location.

This online platform quickly gained popularity as a hub for motivation and encouragement. It served as a virtual community where individuals could come together to prioritize their health and well-being, particularly during a time when physical activity was crucial for maintaining both physical and mental health. The name, "Will Power Sunday Roast," was a nod to the idea that willpower and determination could be as satisfying and nourishing as a hearty Sunday meal.

Each week, I posted new workout routines, exercise challenges, and motivational messages. Participants were encouraged to share their progress, ask questions, and engage in supportive discussions. The sense of camaraderie and shared goals within the community was truly inspiring.

Through "Will Power Sunday Roast," I aimed not only to motivate individuals to engage in physical activity but also to underscore the importance of exercise as a valuable tool in managing diabetes. I shared my own experiences and the positive impact that running, and fitness had on my diabetes management journey, serving as living proof that a healthier, more active lifestyle was achievable.

The initiative also emphasized the power of community in overcoming challenges. Together, we demonstrated that even in the midst of a global pandemic, we could adapt, support one another, and take proactive steps to safeguard our health and well-being. By adapting my routine, and launching the "Will Power Sunday Roast" initiative, I continued to advocate for a healthy and active lifestyle. Through this platform, we formed a supportive community that encouraged individuals to embrace fitness, combat diabetes, and navigate the pandemic with resilience and determination.

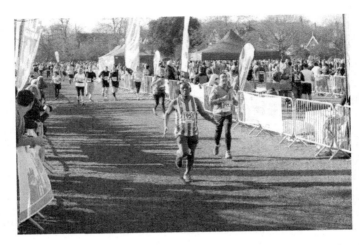

My journey with running has been a testament to the transformative power of exercise in managing and ultimately overcoming diabetes. It has become my mission to share this powerful message of hope and empowerment with others, encouraging and motivating them to embrace physical activity as a means to improve their health, combat diabetes, and foster a profound sense of empowerment.

Through my own experiences, I have witnessed first-hand the positive impact that regular exercise, like running, can have on diabetes management. It's not just about the physical benefits, such as improved weight control, enhanced cardiovascular health, and better blood sugar regulation, although those are certainly crucial. It's also about the mental and emotional well-being that physical activity brings.

Running, in particular, has been a source of tremendous joy and fulfillment in my life. It's an activity that not only strengthens the body but also invigorates the spirit. The endorphin rush, the sense of accomplishment after each run, and the steady progress toward fitness goals all contribute to a positive and resilient mindset. This, in turn, helps individuals facing the challenges of diabetes to approach their condition with determination and optimism.

My goal is to inspire and uplift others on their own journeys toward wellness. I believe that by sharing my story and the lessons I've learned along the way, I can empower individuals to take control of their health and embrace a life filled with vitality and purpose.

Running has transcended being just a personal passion; it has become a powerful tool for advocacy and motivation. I encourage others to lace up their running shoes or engage in any form of physical activity that speaks to them. Whether it's running, walking, swimming, cycling, or dancing, the key is to find an activity that brings joy and aligns with one's goals and abilities.

I firmly believe that every step taken is a victorious step, every mile covered, and every effort made in the realm of physical activity is a step closer to a healthier and more vibrant life. It's a step towards greater resilience, both physically and mentally, and a step towards overcoming the challenges of diabetes.

To those who may be facing diabetes or any other health condition, I offer the message that they are not alone. There is a community of individuals who have walked similar paths, and together, we can provide support, encouragement, and the knowledge that a fulfilling and active life is entirely within reach.

In conclusion, my journey with running has been a journey of transformation, resilience, and empowerment. I am committed to sharing the invaluable lessons I've learned along the way and inspiring others to embrace physical activity as a powerful tool for managing and overcoming diabetes. Running has not only enriched my own life but has become a beacon of hope for all those who dare to take that first victorious steps toward a healthier, more active, and more fulfilling future.

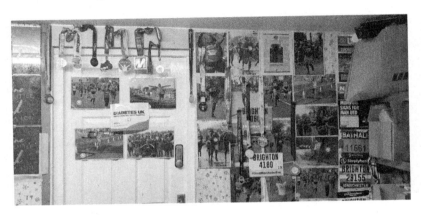

Above: My Hall of fame- Medals!

Tips!

If you're considering starting a running journey, I have a few suggestions to make the process smoother:

1.   Begin with a plan: Create a realistic and attainable plan that includes a balance of walking and jogging intervals. Gradually increase the duration and intensity of your runs over time.

2.   Invest in proper gear: Ensure that you have comfortable and supportive running shoes to minimize the

risk of injuries. Dress appropriately for the weather and consider using running accessories, such as a fitness tracker or running app, to track your progress.

3.   Find a running buddy or join a community: Running with a partner or joining a local running group can provide support, motivation, and accountability. Sharing the journey with others can make it more enjoyable and help you stay committed.

4.   Focus on proper form and technique: Learn about proper running form to avoid injuries and maximize efficiency. Consider seeking guidance from a running coach or attending a running clinic to refine your technique.

5.   Celebrate small victories: Acknowledge and celebrate each milestone, no matter how small. Whether it's running an extra minute or completing a new distance, every achievement is a step forward in your running journey.

Remember, the most important aspect of starting a running journey is to enjoy the process. Embrace the freedom of movement, the rhythm of your footsteps, and the invigorating feeling of the wind against your face. Running has the power to transform your life, both physically and mentally, and I encourage you to take that first step towards a healthier, more empowered you.

Addressing diabetes-related emergencies is crucial for the well-being of individuals with diabetes. Here's a guide on how to handle two common diabetes emergencies: hypoglycemia (low blood sugar) and hyperglycemia (high blood sugar).

Hypoglycemia (Low Blood Sugar):

Hypoglycemia occurs when blood sugar levels drop too low, usually below 70 mg/dL (3.9 mmol/L). It can be caused by excessive insulin, insufficient food, increased physical activity, or other factors. Recognizing and treating hypoglycemia promptly is essential to prevent severe complications.

Recognizing Hypoglycemia:

Common symptoms include shakiness, sweating, irritability, confusion, rapid heartbeat, dizziness, and hunger.
Some individuals may experience tingling sensations in the lips or tongue, headache, or blurred vision.

Steps to Handle Hypoglycemia:

Check Blood Sugar: If you experience symptoms of hypoglycemia, check your blood sugar level immediately if possible.

Consume Fast-Acting Carbohydrates: Consume 15-20 grams of fast-acting carbohydrates to raise your blood sugar quickly. Examples include glucose tablets or gel, four ounces of fruit juice, regular soda (not diet), or a tablespoon of honey or sugar.

Wait and Recheck: Wait 15 minutes after treating the low blood sugar, then recheck your blood sugar levels. If they're still below the target range, repeat the treatment.

Have a Balanced Snack: After stabilizing your blood sugar, have a balanced snack or meal to prevent another drop. Combine carbohydrates with protein or fat for sustained energy.

Notify Others: Let someone close to you know about your hypoglycemia episode and educate them on how to help in case of severe hypoglycemia when you cannot treat yourself.

Wear Medical Alert Identification: Wearing a medical alert bracelet or necklace can inform bystanders and medical professionals about your diabetes in case you are unable to communicate.

Hyperglycemia (High Blood Sugar):

Hyperglycemia occurs when blood sugar levels are consistently above the target range, often exceeding 180 mg/dL (10 mmol/L). It can be caused by insufficient insulin, illness, stress, or poor diabetes management. Long-term hyperglycemia can lead to complications, so it's important to address it promptly.

Recognizing Hyperglycemia:

Common symptoms include excessive thirst, frequent urination, fatigue, blurred vision, slow wound healing, and unexplained weight loss.

Steps to Handle Hyperglycemia:

Check Blood Sugar: Check your blood sugar level to confirm hyperglycemia.

Stay Hydrated: Drink plenty of water to help flush excess glucose from your system. Avoid sugary beverages.

Adjust Medications: If you take diabetes medications, follow your healthcare provider's recommendations for adjusting your medication dosage if needed.

Monitor Ketones: If you have type 1 diabetes, monitor ketones in your urine or blood, especially when blood sugar levels are consistently high. High ketone levels can indicate diabetic ketoacidosis (DKA), a severe and potentially life-threatening condition that requires immediate medical attention.

Review Your Meal Plan: Assess your recent dietary choices and adjust your meal plan to include more balanced, low-glycemic-index foods.

Contact Your Healthcare Provider: If you are unable to lower your blood sugar levels or if you have symptoms of DKA (such as nausea, vomiting, abdominal pain, or fruity breath odor), contact your healthcare provider or seek immediate medical assistance.

It's important to have a diabetes management plan in place and communicate it with loved ones, especially in cases of severe hypoglycemia or hyperglycemia where you may need assistance. Regular monitoring of blood sugar levels and quick action when needed can help individuals with diabetes manage these emergencies effectively.

Chapter 6

Faith as my guide: Finding Strength in God

In the depths of my battle against diabetes, my faith emerged as a steadfast guide, providing unwavering support and strength. It became increasingly clear to me that deepening my faith and spirituality throughout the entire process was not just important but pivotal. My belief in God's healing power became the anchor that kept me grounded and hopeful, even in the face of adversity.

One Bible verse that resonated with me during my journey was Philippians 4:13, which states, "I can do all things through Christ who strengthens me." This verse became a source of inspiration and a reminder that, with faith and determination, I could overcome the challenges posed by diabetes. It reinforced the idea that diabetes did not define my limits; rather, my faith empowered me to take victorious steps over diabetes. My faith journey was a deeply personal one, marked by moments of prayer, reflection, and seeking guidance. I found solace in connecting with a supportive community of believers who understood the importance of faith in times of adversity. Together, we prayed for strength, resilience, and the wisdom to make informed choices about my health.

As I faced the challenges of managing diabetes, my relationship with God became an integral part of my journey.

I found solace and comfort in turning to Him, seeking His guidance and reassurance. Through prayer, meditation, and the study of His Word, I cultivated a profound connection with the Divine, understanding that I was never alone in my struggles.

The Bible became a cherished source of inspiration and encouragement throughout my journey, providing verses that spoke directly to my situation and offered profound reassurance. Here are some of the verses that instilled in me a deep sense of trust and faith, reminding me that God was with me every step of the way:

Isaiah 41:10: "So do not fear, for I am with you; do not be dismayed, for I am your God. I will strengthen you and help you; I will uphold you with my righteous right hand." This verse reminded me that God's presence and strength were always available to me, banishing fear and doubt.

Jeremiah 29:11: "For I know the plans I have for you, declares the Lord, plans for welfare and not for evil, to give you a future and a hope." This verse served as a reminder that God had a purpose for my life, even in the midst of health challenges, and that there was hope for a better future.

Psalm 139:14: "I praise you because I am fearfully and wonderfully made; your works are wonderful, I know that full well." This verse reinforced the idea that despite any physical challenges, my body was a remarkable creation, and I could find wonder and gratitude in it.

Romans 8:28: "And we know that in all things God works for the good of those who love him, who have been called according to his purpose." This verse provided comfort in the belief that even in the face of adversity, God could work all things for my ultimate good.

Proverbs 3:5-6: "Trust in the Lord with all your heart and lean not on your own understanding; in all your ways submit to him, and he will make your paths straight." These verses encouraged me to place my trust in God's wisdom and guidance, even when facing uncertainty.

2 Corinthians 12:9: "But he said to me, 'My grace is sufficient for you, for my power is made perfect in weakness.' Therefore I will boast all the more gladly about my weaknesses, so that Christ's power may rest on me." This verse reminded me that in moments of weakness, God's grace and strength would sustain me.

Matthew 11:28-30: "Come to me, all you who are weary and burdened, and I will give you rest. Take my yoke upon you and learn from me, for I am gentle and humble in heart, and you will find rest for your souls. For my yoke is easy and my burden is light." These words of Jesus offered solace and the promise of rest for my weary spirit.

These verses, among others, became my source of daily inspiration and a constant reminder of God's presence, love, and care in the midst of my journey with diabetes. They strengthened my faith, uplifted my spirit, and guided me through moments of doubt and difficulty.

In the moments of doubt and despair, my faith acted as a beacon of hope. It was through my unwavering belief in God's power that I found the strength to make necessary lifestyle changes, adhere to my medication regimen, and maintain a positive outlook. I recognized that my faith and the practical steps I took to manage my diabetes were not mutually exclusive, but rather intertwined in a harmonious dance of healing and empowerment. I prayed not only for the strength to manage diabetes effectively but also for the possibility of healing. While I understood that healing might not always come in the form of a miraculous cure, I held onto the belief that God's grace and guidance would lead me toward a path of improved health and well-being. Through prayer and meditation, I found moments of clarity and insight. I recognized that my journey with diabetes was not just a physical battle but also a spiritual one—a test of faith, resilience, and personal growth. Diabetes, in its own way, became a catalyst for a deeper connection with my spirituality and a source of strength that propelled me forward.

My faith also played a significant role in managing the emotional and mental aspects of living with diabetes. It provided me with a sense of peace and acceptance, allowing me to navigate the emotional ups and downs that often accompany a chronic condition. I learned to surrender my fears and anxieties to a higher power, trusting that I was not alone in this journey. My faith journey was not without its challenges and doubts. There were moments when I questioned why God had allowed diabetes to enter my life and that of my family members and also whether my faith was strong enough to carry me through. However, I came to understand that faith was not about the absence of doubt but the ability to persevere in spite of it. In the end, my faith became an integral part of my victorious steps over diabetes. It was the unwavering support that sustained me through the darkest days and the source of hope that propelled me toward a future of improved health and well-being. My journey with diabetes was not just a physical battle; it was a spiritual awakening, a testament to the power of faith, and a reminder that even in the face of adversity, we can find strength, resilience, and victorious steps forward.

I cannot overstate the significance of prayer in my journey— it became my lifeline, a direct line of communication with the Divine. In prayer, I found solace and strength, and it played a pivotal role in my victorious steps over diabetes. Here's how it all unfolded.

One of the most profound aspects of prayer is the intimate connection it fostered between me and God. It is a sacred space where I could pour out my heart, expressing my deepest fears, frustrations, and hopes. Just as the Psalms frequently reflect the raw emotions of the psalmists, I, too, laid bare my feelings before the Creator. I knew that God was not distant but an ever-present source of comfort and guidance.

A pivotal aspect of my prayer life was surrender. I learned to surrender my worries and anxieties, acknowledging that there were aspects of diabetes management beyond my control. I drew strength from the Bible verse Matthew 11:28, where Jesus says, "Come to me, all you who are weary and burdened, and I will give you rest." In those moments of surrender, I found peace and the assurance that I was not alone in my journey.

Prayer is also a source of hope. I recalled the miracles of Jesus on healing, like the story of the woman with the issue of blood, who believed that merely touching the hem of Jesus' garment would bring about her healing (Mark 5:25-34). While I understood that miracles might not always manifest in the same way, I held onto the belief that God's divine intervention could lead me toward improved health. Through prayer, I found moments of clarity and insight. It was as if a veil had been lifted, and I could see my journey with diabetes from a broader perspective. I recognized that it was not just a physical battle but a spiritual one—a test of faith, resilience, and personal growth. Prayer allowed me to discern the lessons hidden within the challenges and to find a renewed sense of purpose.

One of the most beautiful aspects of prayer was the sense of being heard and understood. Even when the world felt chaotic and unpredictable, I knew that God was attentive to my prayers. The Bible verse Psalm 34:17-18 resonated deeply with me: "The righteous cry out, and the Lord hears them; he delivers them from all their troubles. The Lord is close to the brokenhearted and saves those who are crushed in spirit." In prayer, I found a safe haven where my troubles could be shared and where I was reminded of God's closeness.

Prayer is not just a religious ritual; it is a source of strength, resilience, and victorious steps forward in my journey with diabetes. It is through prayer that I found the courage to face each day, the wisdom to make informed choices about my health, and the unwavering belief that I could conquer the challenges before me.

In conclusion, prayer is an integral part of my victorious steps over diabetes. It was a lifeline that connected me with the Divine, a source of comfort, and a catalyst for hope and resilience. Just as miracles of healing were woven throughout the Bible, I held onto the belief that through prayer and faith, I could experience my own miracles of improved health and well-being.

I encountered numerous moments that reinforced my faith along this arduous journey. Whether it was a serendipitous meeting with a stranger who offered words of encouragement, a medical breakthrough that aligned perfectly with my needs, or a profound sense of peace during times of uncertainty, these experiences served as reminders of God's presence and His active role in my healing process.

The journey of faith and diabetes intertwined, allowing me to witness the transformative power of God's love and grace. It was through this intertwining that I realized the importance of combining prayer, medication, and exercise. Each component played a vital role in my overall well-being and served as a testament to the holistic approach required in managing diabetes. My faith in God served as the anchor during both the highs and lows of my diabetes journey. It provided me with hope when faced with challenges, reminding me that there was a greater purpose in my struggles. Through prayer, I found solace and direction, and I placed my trust in God's plan for my life.

As I recount the encounters and moments that reinforced my faith, I am driven by a profound desire to inspire and uplift others who may be facing their own battles with diabetes or any other health challenge. It is my hope that by sharing my journey and the role of faith in it, I can encourage individuals to embrace their spirituality and seek solace in God's presence.

Throughout my own journey with diabetes, faith has been an unwavering source of strength and resilience. It's a reminder that, even in the face of adversity, we are not alone. Through prayer, scripture, and a deep connection with God, I have found solace, guidance, and the courage to persevere.

My journey, marked by victorious steps over diabetes, serves as a testament to the power of faith in overcoming life's challenges. By leaning on God's promises and trusting in His divine plan, we can discover the inner strength to face each day with hope and determination.

I invite others to embark on their own faith journey, regardless of the obstacles they may encounter. Embrace the comforting words of scripture, draw strength from prayer, and find solace in the knowledge that God is with you every step of the way.

It is my fervent belief that through faith, we can rise above the challenges of diabetes and emerge stronger, more resilient, and empowered to take control of our health and well-being. Just as I have experienced victorious steps in my journey, I wholeheartedly believe that others can, too, by placing their trust in God and finding inspiration in their spirituality.

Tips!
The relationship between faith and diabetes can be profound and multifaceted. Many individuals living with diabetes find that their faith plays a significant role in how they cope with

the condition and make sense of its challenges. Here are some ways in which faith can intersect with diabetes:

Emotional Support: Faith can provide emotional strength and resilience when dealing with the daily demands and potential frustrations of diabetes management. Believing in a higher power can offer comfort and a sense of purpose during difficult times.

Coping Mechanism: Faith can serve as a coping mechanism for handling stress and anxiety associated with diabetes. Prayer, meditation, or spiritual practices can help individuals find peace and inner strength.

Community and Support: Many religious communities offer a sense of belonging and support for individuals with diabetes. Supportive fellow congregants or community members can provide encouragement and understanding.

Guidance on Lifestyle Choices: Some faith traditions emphasize principles of healthy living, which can align with diabetes management. These principles may include moderation in eating, regular physical activity, and avoiding harmful substances.

Rituals and Fasting: For some people, religious rituals and fasting are integral aspects of their faith. These practices may require adjustments in diabetes management, such as careful planning and consultation with healthcare professionals.

Hope and Resilience: Faith can instill a sense of hope and resilience, encouraging individuals to persevere in their diabetes management efforts and maintain a positive outlook.

Decision-Making: Faith can influence healthcare decision-making. Some individuals may seek guidance from their religious leaders or rely on prayer when making choices about treatment or lifestyle changes.

Community Resources: Faith-based organizations often provide resources and programs related to health and wellness, including diabetes education and support groups.

It's important to note that the relationship between faith and diabetes is highly personal and can vary widely from person to person. Some individuals may find that their faith greatly enhances their diabetes management, while others may have a more limited or different experience.

If you have diabetes and wish to explore the connection between your faith and your condition, consider speaking with a healthcare provider or diabetes educator who is sensitive to your spiritual needs. They can offer guidance on integrating your faith into your diabetes management plan and addressing any specific concerns or questions you may have.

Chapter 7

A Legacy of Diabetes: Navigating Family History

Within the intricate tapestry of my family's health history, the presence of diabetes weaves a thread that cannot be ignored. It is a condition that has left an indelible mark on our lives, shaping our family dynamics and inspiring us to find effective strategies for managing this chronic illness. In the early 2010s to 2015, a significant shift occurred as five of my siblings received the life-altering diagnosis of diabetes. This marked a turning point, both individually and collectively, as we grappled with the impact of this condition and sought ways to navigate the challenges it presented.

Amidst this familial shift, my mother emerged as a pillar of strength. She had been living with diabetes for over 24 years, and her journey became a guiding light for all of us. Despite the obstacles she faced, she exemplified resilience and determination in managing her diabetes. Through her commitment to regular exercise, a balanced diet, and consistent self-care, she demonstrated that it was possible to maintain control over this condition and live a fulfilling life.

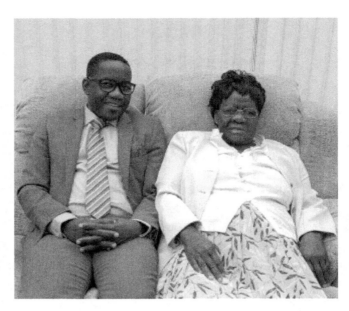

With my Mother

However, our family history also bore witness to the devastating consequences of diabetes. We mourned the loss of my uncle and aunt, both of whom succumbed to this relentless condition. Their passing served as a stark reminder that diabetes should never be taken lightly, even for those who appear fit and healthy. It underscored the importance of vigilance and regular check-ups, regardless of age or perceived well-being.

The diagnosis of multiple siblings within a short span of time created a sense of urgency and heightened awareness within our family. We realized that our genetic predisposition to diabetes demanded our attention and proactive measures. We embarked on a collective journey of education, support, and mutual understanding.

The impact of diabetes on our family extended far beyond the physical manifestations of the condition. Emotionally, we experienced a range of emotions, from fear and uncertainty to a deep sense of responsibility. Each of us grappled with our own fears and concerns, as we witnessed the profound effects that diabetes had on our loved ones.

As we navigated this shared journey, we became a united front, seeking to support one another in any way possible. We attended educational seminars together, joined support groups, and shared valuable resources and information. Our family bond grew stronger as we realized that we were not alone in facing the challenges of diabetes.

Through this collective experience, we learned the importance of early detection and proactive measures in managing diabetes. We discovered that knowledge is power, and that understanding our family history provided crucial insight into our individual risks. Armed with this knowledge, we were able to make informed decisions about our own health and take the necessary steps to prevent or manage diabetes.

Our family's history of diabetes served as a clear indicator of our increased risk. Armed with this knowledge, we understood the need for proactive measures to monitor our health. We encourage everyone, especially those with a family history of diabetes, to undergo regular screenings and check-ups to catch any potential signs of the condition at its earliest stages.

Education became a cornerstone of our diabetes management approach. We immersed ourselves in learning about the intricacies of diabetes, understanding its impact on our bodies, and the steps necessary to control it. We attended seminars, workshops, and engaged in discussions with healthcare professionals who provided valuable insights and guidance. This knowledge empowered us to make informed decisions about our lifestyle choices, diet, and exercise routines.

Developing healthy habits is another vital aspect of our journey. We recognized that small, consistent changes could make a significant difference in managing diabetes. We focused on adopting a balanced diet, emphasizing whole foods, fruits, vegetables, and lean proteins, while reducing our intake of processed sugars and unhealthy fats. Regular physical activity, like walking, jogging, or engaging in sports, has become an integral part of our daily routine. Exercise not only helped regulate blood sugar levels but also promoted overall well-being and strengthened our bodies.

Support played a pivotal role in our diabetes management. We leaned on each other for encouragement, motivation, and shared experiences. Through support groups, both online and offline, we connected with others facing similar challenges. These networks provided a safe space to express our concerns, share strategies, and celebrate victories. We found solace in knowing that we were not alone on this journey and that there was a wealth of knowledge and support available to us.

Our family's experience also taught us the importance of maintaining a positive mindset. Diabetes can present daily obstacles and frustrations, but approaching it with a positive attitude can make a world of difference. We focused on gratitude, finding joy in the small victories, and celebrating progress along the way. By cultivating a positive mindset, we were able to navigate challenges with resilience, determination, and a belief that we had the power to overcome them.

Throughout our collective journey, we discovered that managing diabetes is not just about physical health; it encompasses mental, emotional, and spiritual well-being as well. We found solace in prayer, meditation, and nurturing our spiritual connections. We recognized the importance of self-care, carving out moments for relaxation, and engaging in activities that brought us joy and peace.

In this chapter, we have shared the valuable lessons we learned from our family's history of diabetes. These lessons have become guiding principles that have transformed our lives and empowered us to take control of our health. Through early detection, education, healthy habits, support networks, and a positive mindset, we have paved the way for a brighter, healthier future, not only for ourselves but also for future generations.

Tips!

Checking your family history for diabetes is an essential step in understanding your risk factors and taking proactive measures to manage your health. Here are some tips to help you effectively gather information about diabetes in your family:

Start Conversations: Initiate open and honest conversations with your family members. Talk to your parents, siblings, grandparents, aunts, uncles, and cousins about their health histories. Encourage them to share any information related to diabetes diagnoses within the family.

Create a Family Health Tree: Consider creating a family health tree or diagram that includes information about diabetes and other chronic conditions. This visual representation can help you see patterns and identify potential risk factors more easily.

Ask Specific Questions: Be sure to ask specific questions when discussing family history. Inquire about the age at which relatives were diagnosed with diabetes, the type of diabetes (type 1 or type 2), and any related complications or comorbidities.

Document Information: Keep detailed records of the information you gather. Note the names of family members, their relationships to you, and their diabetes-related details. You can use a notebook, a family health history form, or even digital tools to organize this information.

Consider Both Sides: Remember to collect information from both sides of your family—maternal and paternal. Diabetes can be influenced by genetic factors from both sides, so a comprehensive family health history should cover all relatives.

Include Extended Family: Don't limit your inquiry to immediate family members. Extended family, such as cousins, aunts, and uncles, can also provide valuable insights into your family's diabetes history.

Seek Medical Records: If possible, request access to medical records or documents that contain health-related information about family members. These records may provide additional details about diabetes diagnoses and management.

Use Online Resources: Utilize online tools and resources that can help you organize and analyze your family health history. Some websites and apps offer templates and guidance for creating comprehensive family health trees.

Update Regularly: Family health histories can change over time as new information becomes available or as relatives develop health conditions. Make it a habit to update your family health tree periodically.

Share with Healthcare Providers: Share your family health history with your healthcare provider during regular check-ups. They can use this information to assess your risk and develop a personalized plan for diabetes prevention or management.

Understanding your family history of diabetes is a proactive step towards managing your health and reducing your risk of developing the condition. By gathering and documenting this information, you can work with healthcare professionals to make informed decisions about your health and well-being.

Diabetes prevalence varies by race and ethnicity globally, and it's important to note that these patterns can differ significantly from one country or region to another. Here's a general overview of diabetes prevalence by race/ethnicity on a global scale:

1. Global Diabetes Prevalence by Region:

Western Pacific Region: This region, which includes countries like China, Japan, and Australia, has a significant burden of diabetes. China, in particular, has one of the largest populations of people with diabetes in the world.

Southeast Asia: Countries in Southeast Asia, such as India and Indonesia, have seen a rapid increase in diabetes prevalence due to factors like urbanization, changing diets, and sedentary lifestyles.

Middle East and North Africa: This region has a high prevalence of diabetes, with countries like Saudi Arabia and Kuwait having some of the highest rates in the world. Genetic factors and a rise in obesity have contributed to this trend.

North America: In the United States and Canada, diabetes prevalence varies among different racial and ethnic groups. Indigenous populations and certain minority groups, such as African Americans and Hispanics, have higher rates of diabetes compared to the general population.

Sub-Saharan Africa: While diabetes prevalence has historically been lower in sub-Saharan Africa compared to other regions, it is on the rise due to factors like urbanization, dietary changes, and increasing obesity rates.

Europe: Diabetes prevalence varies across European countries, with some countries in Eastern Europe experiencing higher rates. Eastern European countries like Russia and Ukraine have seen an increase in diabetes prevalence.

2. Diabetes Prevalence by Race/Ethnicity Globally:

Indigenous Populations: Indigenous populations, including Native Americans in the United States and Canada, as well as Aboriginal and Torres Strait Islander peoples in Australia, often have a higher prevalence of diabetes compared to non-indigenous populations.

African Descent: People of African descent, both on the African continent and in the African diaspora, can have a higher risk of diabetes. Factors such as genetics and socio-economic disparities may contribute to this risk.

South Asian Descent: South Asian populations, including those from India, Pakistan, Bangladesh, and Sri Lanka, have a higher risk of developing diabetes, often at a younger age and lower BMI, due to genetic and lifestyle factors.

It's important to emphasize that these patterns are not uniform within or between countries. Diabetes prevalence can be influenced by a combination of genetic factors, lifestyle choices (such as diet and physical activity), healthcare access, and socio-economic status. Public health efforts and interventions are essential to address and manage diabetes within these diverse populations. Therefore, diabetes prevention and management strategies need to be tailored to the specific needs and risk factors of different racial and ethnic groups in various regions of the world.

Chapter 8

Empowering Others: Advice for People with Diabetes

Now, as we conclude, I want to leave you with some essential tips that can guide you on your own journey of managing diabetes and living a vibrant, fulfilling life. I want to encourage every reader who has experienced the weight of diabetes to find their own path to triumph. Each journey will be unique, but the principles remain the same—faith, perseverance, and a commitment to a healthy lifestyle.

Self-management is a crucial aspect of effectively managing diabetes. It involves knowledge, action, and accountability to maintain blood sugar levels within a target range, prevent complications, and improve overall well-being. Here's a breakdown of self-management in diabetes with a focus on knowledge, action, and accountability:

1. Knowledge: Understanding Diabetes: Educate yourself about diabetes, its types (e.g., type 1, type 2, gestational diabetes), and its impact on the body. Understanding the basics of diabetes is essential for effective self-management.

Blood Glucose Monitoring: Learn how to monitor your blood glucose levels using a blood glucose meter or continuous glucose monitor (CGM). Understand what your target blood sugar range should be and when and how often to check your levels.

Carbohydrate Counting: Learn how to count carbohydrates in your meals and snacks. Carbohydrate counting is crucial for dosing insulin or managing medications effectively.

Medications and Insulin: If prescribed medications or insulin, understand how they work, when and how to take them, and potential side effects. Comply with your healthcare provider's recommendations for medication management.

Diet and Nutrition: Get guidance from a registered dietitian to develop a personalized meal plan. Learn how different foods affect your blood sugar and how to make healthy food choices.

Physical Activity: Understand the importance of regular physical activity in diabetes management. Learn how exercise affects blood sugar levels and develop a suitable exercise routine.

2. Action:

Healthy Eating: Make sure you look after yourself and eat properly to avoid the chances of developing diabetes and other related problems such as high blood pressure. Remember that a balanced diet, rich in fruits, vegetables, lean proteins, and whole grains, is crucial for maintaining optimal health. By nourishing your body with wholesome foods, you provide it with the nutrients it needs to thrive. Follow your meal plan, focusing on a balanced diet that includes lean proteins, whole grains, fruits, vegetables, and healthy fats. Monitor portion sizes and limit sugary and high-carbohydrate foods.

Regular Physical Activity: Incorporate regular physical activity into your daily routine. Aim for at least 150 minutes of moderate-intensity aerobic activity per week, along with strength training exercises. The benefits of exercise in managing diabetes are numerous. Physical activity helps regulate blood sugar levels, improves cardiovascular health, boosts mood, reduces stress, and contributes to overall well-being. Find activities that you enjoy, whether it's walking, swimming, cycling, or dancing, and make exercise a consistent part of your routine. Commit to a fitness regime that works for you. It may be running, walking, swimming, or any other form of exercise that ignites your passion. Find joy in movement, and let it be your ally in managing diabetes and improving your overall well-being.

Medication Management: Take your medications or insulin as prescribed by your healthcare provider. Follow the recommended dosage and timing carefully.

Blood Glucose Monitoring: Regularly check your blood sugar levels as advised by your healthcare provider. Use the results to make informed decisions about your meals, physical activity, and medication.

Stress Management: Practice stress-reduction techniques like mindfulness, meditation, or deep breathing exercises. Stress can affect blood sugar levels, so managing it is essential.

Hydration: Stay well-hydrated by drinking plenty of water. Limit sugary beverages and monitor their impact on your blood sugar.

Regular Check-ups: Attend regular check-ups with your healthcare provider to monitor your diabetes control, assess complications, and adjust your treatment plan as needed.

3. Accountability:

Keep Records: Maintain a diabetes journal to track your blood sugar levels, meals, medications, physical activity, and any symptoms or unusual events. Keeping records can help identify patterns and areas for improvement.

Set Goals: Work with your healthcare provider to establish realistic goals for diabetes management. These goals can be related to blood sugar targets, weight management, or other aspects of diabetes care.

Review Progress: Regularly review your progress with your healthcare team. Discuss any challenges you face, ask questions, and seek guidance on adjustments to your treatment plan. Keep regular appointments to check your eyes, kidneys, feet, and other vital organs affected by diabetes. Regular screenings and check-ups play a crucial role in detecting and managing potential complications. By prioritizing these appointments, you ensure that any issues are identified and addressed promptly, minimizing the impact on your overall health.

Engage in Support: Remember, you are not alone. Reach out, seek support, and embark on this journey with a renewed sense of hope and empowerment. Together, we can overcome the obstacles and embrace a brighter, healthier future. Join support groups. Connecting with others who share similar experiences can be immensely beneficial in managing diabetes. Support groups provide a sense of belonging, understanding, and empathy. They offer a platform to share insights, challenges, and successes, and provide a source of encouragement and motivation. You are not alone in this journey, and surrounding yourself with a supportive community can make a significant difference in your well-being. Join diabetes support groups or seek support from friends and family. Sharing your experiences and challenges with others who understand can provide motivation and accountability.

Self-Advocacy: Be an advocate for your own health. Ask questions, seek second opinions if necessary, and communicate openly with your healthcare provider about your concerns and preferences.

Family History: Check your family history to see if anyone in your lineage has diabetes. This can serve as an indicator of your own potential risk. Understanding your family's health history allows you to take proactive steps in managing your well-being and seeking early interventions if needed. Knowledge is power, and by being aware of your family's health background, you can make informed choices about your own health.

Signs and symptoms: Be vigilant for signs of diabetes, such as excessive thirst, frequent urination, unexplained weight loss, or extreme fatigue. These may be potential indicators that further investigation is necessary. Your body often communicates its needs and concerns, so it is essential to listen and be proactive in addressing any potential health issues.

Seek professional help. If you suspect you may have diabetes or if you have been diagnosed with the condition, it is crucial to seek the guidance of healthcare professionals. They possess the knowledge and expertise to help you manage your diabetes effectively. Regular consultations with doctors, nurses, dietitians, and other healthcare professionals can provide invaluable support on your journey.

Remember to pray. Faith in God can provide solace, strength, and comfort during the challenges of living with diabetes. Believe in the power of prayer and trust that God is a healer. "But He was wounded for our transgressions, He was bruised for our iniquities: the chastisement of our peace was upon Him; and with His stripes, we are healed" (Isaiah 53:5, KJV). Seek spiritual guidance, find peace in your connection with the divine, and draw strength from your faith.

Above all, never lose sight of the fact that you are not alone in this fight. There are countless individuals who have conquered diabetes, defying the odds and reclaiming their lives. They stand as beacons of inspiration, reminding us that victory is possible, and that we have the power to shape our own destinies.

Medication

There are several types of diabetes medications available to help manage blood sugar levels in people with diabetes. The choice of medication depends on the type of diabetes a person has (type 1 or type 2), individual needs, and other factors. Here are some common categories of diabetes medications:

For Type 1 Diabetes:

Insulin: People with type 1 diabetes typically require insulin therapy to replace the hormone their body does not produce. There are various types of insulin, including rapid-acting, short-acting, intermediate-acting, and long-acting, which are used in different combinations to mimic the body's natural insulin release.

For Type 2 Diabetes:

Metformin: Metformin is often the first-line medication for type 2 diabetes. It helps reduce glucose production by the liver and improves insulin sensitivity in the body.

Sulfonylureas: These medications stimulate the pancreas to release more insulin. Examples include glyburide, glipizide, and glimepiride.

Dipeptidyl Peptidase-4 (DPP-4) Inhibitors: DPP-4 inhibitors, such as sitagliptin and saxagliptin, increase insulin release and reduce blood sugar levels.

SGLT2 Inhibitors: Sodium-glucose cotransporter-2 (SGLT2) inhibitors, like empagliflozin and dapagliflozin, work by reducing glucose reabsorption in the kidneys and promoting its excretion in urine.

GLP-1 Receptor Agonists: Glucagon-like peptide-1 (GLP-1) receptor agonists, such as liraglutide and exenatide, increase insulin secretion, slow digestion, and reduce appetite.

Thiazolidinediones (TZDs): TZDs, like pioglitazone and rosiglitazone, improve insulin sensitivity in the body's cells.

Alpha-Glucosidase Inhibitors: These medications slow down the digestion of carbohydrates and reduce glucose absorption in the intestines. Acarbose is an example.

Meglitinides: Meglitinides, such as repaglinide and nateglinide, stimulate the pancreas to produce insulin, but they have a shorter duration of action than sulfonylureas.

Basal Insulin: Some people with type 2 diabetes may require basal insulin in addition to oral medications to provide a steady background level of insulin.

Combination Medications: Some medications combine two or more of the classes mentioned above to provide a synergistic effect and simplify treatment.

It's important to note that the choice of diabetes medication is highly individualized, and the treatment plan should be determined by a healthcare provider based on the patient's specific needs, medical history, and blood sugar control goals. Lifestyle factors, such as diet and physical activity, also play a crucial role in diabetes management. Regular monitoring of blood sugar levels and close communication with a healthcare team are essential for effective diabetes management.
Embrace the responsibility of looking after your diabetes. Remember that managing diabetes is possible. With the right

mindset, education, support, and proactive self-care, you can live a fulfilling life while effectively managing your condition. Empower yourself with knowledge, make informed choices, and prioritize your health and well-being.

Remember, setbacks may occur, and relapses can happen. But let those moments serve as reminders of your strength and resilience. Don't let them define you. Instead, use them as opportunities for growth and renewal. Learn from them, adjust your approach if needed, and keep moving forward with determination.

I hope that the stories, experiences, and insights shared have ignited a flame of hope and empowerment within you. The journey of triumphing over diabetes has been a transformational one. As I look back on my fight against this relentless condition, I am filled with a profound sense of gratitude for the lessons learned and the positive outcomes that have emerged from the depths of adversity. Throughout these chapters, we have explored the depths of living with diabetes, the challenges it presents, and the triumphs that can be achieved through faith, resilience, and a proactive approach to self-care. Throughout these chapters, I have shared the story of my life before diabetes, the diagnosis that shook me to my core, the struggles I faced when I resisted professional advice, and the battles I fought against the effects of diabetes. I have recounted the turning point when I embraced faith and fitness, and how running became a catalyst for reclaiming my health and defying the limitations of the condition.

But this journey is not just about me. It is about every individual who faces the challenges of diabetes and yearns for victory. It is about finding the strength within us, to rise above adversity and to believe in our ability to make positive changes. Embrace faith, whatever that means to you. Whether it is through prayer, meditation, or a deep connection to something greater than yourself, faith can provide solace, hope, and the belief that you can overcome any obstacle.

As we conclude this journey together, I want to remind you that you are capable, strong, and deserving of a vibrant, healthy life. Diabetes may be a part of your story, but it does not define you. Let the lessons, strategies, and insights shared within these pages guide you on your path to success. Embrace the power of faith, harness the strength within, and forge ahead with confidence and determination. I want to encourage every reader who has experienced the weight of diabetes to find their own path to triumph. Each journey will be unique, but the principles remain the same—faith, perseverance, and a commitment to a healthy lifestyle. Effective self-management in diabetes is a lifelong commitment. By acquiring knowledge, taking proactive actions, and being accountable for your health, you can optimize your diabetes management, reduce the risk of complications, and enjoy a healthier and more fulfilling life. Remember that you don't have to navigate this journey alone; your healthcare team is there to provide guidance and support.

May this book serve as a guiding light, offering insights, encouragement, and practical advice to those who walk the path of triumph over diabetes. May it inspire you to take charge of your health, embrace faith, and cultivate a lifestyle that nurtures your well-being. May you find the strength within yourself to overcome any obstacle and to live a life of victory over diabetes.

For both you and me, the journey toward triumph over diabetes is an ongoing one, marked by victorious steps along the way. I'm grateful to have shared a part of this journey with you. As we continue on this path, may you discover your own victorious steps, leading you toward triumph over diabetes, and may your future be filled with health, joy, and abundant blessings. May you find your own path to triumph and create a future filled with health, joy, and abundant blessings.

Resources

People with diabetes need to manage their condition through regular monitoring and adopting a healthy lifestyle. Here are some necessary checks and measures for people with diabetes:

Blood Glucose Monitoring:

Regularly check blood glucose levels as recommended by your healthcare provider. This can be done using a blood glucose meter or continuous glucose monitoring (CGM) system.

Hemoglobin A1c Test:

Get an A1c test every three to six months to assess your long-term blood glucose control. The target A1c level may vary based on your individual circumstances, but generally, it should be below 7%.

Blood Pressure Monitoring:

Regularly check and control your blood pressure to reduce the risk of heart disease and kidney problems. Aim for a target blood pressure of 130/80 mm Hg or as advised by your healthcare provider.

Cholesterol Level Monitoring:

Have your cholesterol levels checked regularly to manage cardiovascular risk factors. Pay attention to LDL ("bad") cholesterol levels.

Kidney Function Tests:

Regularly monitor kidney function through tests like serum creatinine and estimated glomerular filtration rate (eGFR) to detect any signs of kidney damage.

Eye Exams:

Schedule regular eye exams with an eye specialist (ophthalmologist) to monitor for diabetic retinopathy, a common complication of diabetes.

Foot Exams:

Regularly inspect your feet for any signs of wounds, blisters, or sores. Consult a podiatrist for a comprehensive foot exam at least annually.

Dental Check-ups:

Maintain good oral hygiene and have regular dental check-ups, as diabetes can increase the risk of gum disease.

Immunizations:

Stay up-to-date on vaccinations, including the annual flu shot and vaccines for pneumonia and hepatitis B, as recommended by your healthcare provider.

Medication Management:

Take prescribed medications as directed by your healthcare provider. Follow the prescribed insulin or oral medications and report any side effects or concerns.

Diet and Nutrition:

Work with a registered dietitian or nutritionist to develop a balanced meal plan that helps manage blood sugar levels. Monitor carbohydrate intake and make healthy food choices.

Physical Activity:

Engage in regular physical activity, as recommended by your healthcare provider. Exercise can help improve insulin sensitivity and overall health.

Stress Management:

Learn stress-reduction techniques such as mindfulness, meditation, or yoga, as stress can affect blood sugar levels.

Weight Management:

Maintain a healthy weight or work towards achieving a healthy weight if needed. Weight management is important for blood sugar control.

Medication and Insulin Adjustments:

Be prepared to adjust medications or insulin doses based on your blood glucose levels and under the guidance of your healthcare provider.

Education and Support:

Stay informed about diabetes management through education programs and support groups. Knowledge and a strong support system are essential for long-term success.

Always consult your healthcare provider for personalized guidance on managing your diabetes, as individual needs and goals may vary. Regular communication with your healthcare team is crucial for effectively managing diabetes and preventing complications.

Terminology

Diabetes is a complex medical condition, and it has its own set of terminology and jargon that are commonly used in the field. Here are some key terms and phrases used in diabetes:

Diabetes Mellitus: The formal medical name for diabetes, often just referred to as "diabetes." It's a chronic condition that affects how your body processes glucose (sugar) in the blood.

Glucose: A type of sugar that comes from the foods we eat and is used by the body for energy. In diabetes, the body has trouble regulating blood glucose levels.

Blood Glucose: The amount of glucose in your bloodstream at a given time. Measured in milligrams per deciliter (mg/dL) in the United States or millimoles per liter (mmol/L) in other countries.

Hyperglycemia: High blood glucose levels, a common problem in diabetes when the body doesn't have enough insulin or can't use it properly.

Hypoglycemia: Low blood glucose levels, often referred to as a "hypo." It can occur when there's too much insulin in the bloodstream or when a person with diabetes hasn't eaten enough.

Insulin: A hormone produced by the pancreas that helps regulate blood glucose levels by allowing glucose to enter cells for energy. People with type 1 diabetes need insulin injections or an insulin pump, while some with type 2 diabetes also require insulin.

Type 1 Diabetes: An autoimmune condition where the body's immune system mistakenly attacks and destroys insulin-producing cells in the pancreas. People with type 1 diabetes require lifelong insulin therapy.

Type 2 Diabetes: A metabolic disorder where the body becomes resistant to insulin or doesn't produce enough of it. Lifestyle changes, medications, and sometimes insulin are used to manage type 2 diabetes.

Prediabetes: A condition where blood glucose levels are higher than normal but not yet in the diabetes range. It's a warning sign that type 2 diabetes may develop if not managed.

A1c (HbA1c): A blood test that measures average blood glucose levels over the past 2-3 months. It's a key tool in diabetes management.

Carbohydrate Counting: A method used by people with diabetes to track the amount of carbohydrates in their meals, which helps determine insulin dosage.

Glycemic Index (GI): A measure of how quickly a carbohydrate-containing food raises blood glucose levels. Foods with a high GI cause a rapid spike in blood sugar.

Continuous Glucose Monitoring (CGM): A device that measures blood glucose levels continuously throughout the day and night, providing real-time data and trends.

Basal Insulin: The insulin needed to maintain blood glucose levels during periods of fasting, such as between meals and overnight.

Bolus Insulin: Additional insulin taken to cover the rise in blood glucose levels after eating. It's calculated based on the carbohydrate content of the meal.

Honeymoon Phase: A period shortly after the diagnosis of type 1 diabetes when the pancreas may still produce some insulin.

Ketoacidosis (DKA): A life-threatening complication of untreated or under-treated diabetes, often seen in type 1 diabetes. It results in high blood ketone levels and requires immediate medical attention.

Hemoglobin A1c (HbA1c): Another term for A1c, a blood test that reflects average blood glucose levels over several months.

Complications: Long-term health issues that can result from uncontrolled diabetes, including neuropathy, retinopathy, nephropathy, and cardiovascular problems.

Diabetes Educator: A healthcare professional who specializes in helping individuals manage their diabetes through education and support.

These are just some of the many terms and phrases used in the field of diabetes. Managing diabetes effectively involves understanding and using this terminology to make informed decisions about diet, medication, exercise, and overall health.

Support Groups in United Kingdom

Support groups for diabetes in the UK provide a valuable resource for individuals living with diabetes and their families. These groups offer emotional support, information sharing, and a sense of community for those affected by diabetes. Here are some prominent diabetes support groups in the UK:

Diabetes UK: Diabetes UK is the leading charity organization dedicated to diabetes in the UK. They offer a range of resources, support, and information on managing diabetes. They also have local groups and communities across the country.

Website: Diabetes UK

JDRF (Juvenile Diabetes Research Foundation): JDRF is a charity that focuses on type 1 diabetes and funds research to find a cure. They also provide support and information for people with type 1 diabetes and their families.

Website: JDRF UK

NHS Diabetes Support Groups: The NHS often organizes diabetes support groups at the local level. These groups can be a valuable resource for connecting with others who have diabetes.

Website: Check with your local NHS services or your healthcare provider for information on local support groups.

Diabetes.co.uk Forum: Diabetes.co.uk offers an online community and forum where people with diabetes can connect, share experiences, and seek advice.

Website: Diabetes.co.uk Forum

Diabetes Support on HealthUnlocked: HealthUnlocked is an online platform that hosts various health-related communities, including diabetes support groups. You can find and join discussions on different aspects of diabetes management.

Website: Diabetes Support on HealthUnlocked

Diabetes Peer Support Groups: Some local communities and hospitals may host peer support groups specifically for people with diabetes. Check with your healthcare provider or local community centers for information on any such groups in your area.

Facebook Groups: There are numerous Facebook groups dedicated to diabetes, where you can connect with others, ask questions, and find support.
Example: "Diabetes UK Support Group" on Facebook

Meetup: The Meetup platform often hosts diabetes support groups and events in various cities across the UK. It's worth checking for diabetes-related Meetup groups in your area.
Website: Meetup

When seeking a diabetes support group, it's essential to find one that suits your specific needs, whether you have type 1 or type 2 diabetes, are a caregiver, or are looking for online or in-person support. These groups can provide valuable insights, motivation, and a sense of community to help you manage diabetes effectively

American Diabetes Association (ADA):
Website: diabetes.org
The ADA offers comprehensive information on diabetes, including prevention, management, and advocacy resources.

National Institute of Diabetes and Digestive and Kidney Diseases (NIDDK):
Website: niddk.nih.gov

NIDDK provides research-based information on diabetes, related conditions, and treatment options.

Diabetes Forecast Magazine:
Website: diabetesforecast.org
Diabetes Forecast offers articles, recipes, and lifestyle tips for diabetes management.

CDC - Diabetes:
Website: cdc.gov/diabetes
The Centers for Disease Control and Prevention provides information on diabetes prevention, awareness campaigns, and educational materials.
Support Communities:

TuDiabetes:
Website: forum.tudiabetes.org
TuDiabetes is an online community where individuals with diabetes can connect, share experiences, and seek support.

Diabetes Daily:
Website: diabetesdaily.com
Diabetes Daily offers forums, articles, and resources for people living with diabetes.

Diabetes Forecast Community:
Website: community.diabetes.org
This community forum is part of the American Diabetes Association and provides a platform for discussions and support.
Beyond Type 1:
Website: beyondtype1.org

Beyond Type 1 is a community for those impacted by type 1 diabetes, offering stories, resources, and advocacy initiatives.

Research and Clinical Trials:
ClinicalTrials.gov:
Website: clinicaltrials.gov
Search for clinical trials related to diabetes and find opportunities to participate in research studies.

Diabetes Research Institute Foundation:
Website: diabetesresearch.org
This organization funds research into curing diabetes and improving treatment options.

Apps and Tools:
There are many useful apps available for people with diabetes that can help with various aspects of diabetes management, such as blood glucose tracking, carb counting, medication reminders, and lifestyle monitoring. Here are some popular diabetes management apps:

MyFitnessPal:
MyFitnessPal is a comprehensive nutrition and exercise tracking app. It's useful for people with diabetes to track their meals, count carbohydrates, and monitor physical activity.

Glucose Buddy:
Glucose Buddy is a user-friendly app for tracking blood glucose levels, insulin, and medications. It also provides charts and graphs to visualize trends.
MySugr:

MySugr offers a diabetes logbook with an easy-to-use interface. It includes features like reminders, data analysis, and the ability to share reports with healthcare providers.

BG Monitor Diabetes:
BG Monitor Diabetes allows users to record blood glucose levels, medications, **meals, and activities. It provides graphs and reports to help analyze patterns.**

Diabetes:M:
Diabetes:M is a comprehensive diabetes management app that tracks blood sugar, insulin, medications, diet, and activity. It offers data export and integration with fitness trackers.

Glucosio:
Glucosio is an open-source diabetes app that helps users track blood sugar levels, medication, and lifestyle factors. It's free and ad-free.

Fooducate:
Fooducate is a nutrition app that can help people with diabetes make healthier food choices by providing information about the nutritional content of various foods.

Carb Manager:
Carb Manager is a carb-counting app that can be helpful for those who need to manage their carbohydrate intake, which is important for blood sugar control.

Dexcom G6 Mobile:

If you use the Dexcom G6 continuous glucose monitoring (CGM) system, this app allows you to monitor your glucose levels in real-time on your smartphone.

Insulin Calculator Apps:
Some insulin pumps come with companion apps that can help calculate insulin doses based on blood sugar levels and carbohydrate intake.

Apple Health and Google Fit:
These built-in health apps on many smartphones allow users to track various health metrics, including blood glucose, activity, and nutrition.

One Drop:
One Drop offers a comprehensive diabetes management platform with features like blood glucose tracking, medication management, and a community for support.

Sugar Sense:
Sugar Sense is an app designed to help users manage diabetes by tracking blood sugar levels, medications, and food intake.

Medisafe:

Medisafe is a medication management app that can help people with diabetes remember to take their medications on time.

Diabetes Forecast Magazine:

The Diabetes Forecast Magazine app provides articles, recipes, and tips for living well with diabetes.

MyFitnessPal:

Website: myfitnesspal.com

MyFitnessPal offers a mobile app to track food intake, exercise, and manage weight, which can be useful for diabetes management.

Glucose Buddy:

Website: glucosebuddy.com

Glucose Buddy is a diabetes management app for tracking blood sugar levels and related data.

Before choosing an app, consider your specific needs and preferences. Some apps may sync with wearable devices or integrate with electronic health records, while others focus on specific aspects of diabetes management. Consult with your healthcare provider to determine which app(s) might be most suitable for your diabetes management plan. Additionally, ensure that the app you choose complies with your privacy and data security preferences.

Nutrition and Diet:

Choose My Plate:

Website: choosemyplate.gov

This resource by the USDA offers dietary guidelines, meal planning tools, and nutrition information.

Diabetes Food Hub:

Website: diabetesfoodhub.org

The Diabetes Food Hub provides recipes, meal plans, and nutrition tips specifically designed for people with diabetes.

Books:

"The Diabetes Code" by Dr. Jason Fung:

A book that explores the root causes of type 2 diabetes and strategies for reversing it.

"Think Like a Pancreas" by Gary Scheiner:

A guide to understanding diabetes management, including insulin therapy and blood sugar control.

Others:

Diabetes UK:

Website: diabetes.org.uk

Diabetes UK offers information and support for people with diabetes in the United Kingdom.

International Diabetes Federation (IDF):

Website: idf.org

IDF is a global organization working to promote diabetes care, prevention, and awareness worldwide.

Diabetes Australia:

Website: diabetesaustralia.com.au

Provides information and resources for diabetes management in Australia.

These resources cover a wide range of topics related to diabetes, from general education to support communities and tools for managing the condition effectively. Remember to consult with your healthcare provider for personalized advice and guidance on diabetes management.

Printed in Great Britain
by Amazon

28191664R00086